FED UP
The Food Forces That Make You Fat, Sick and Poor

by Brett Silverstein

SOUTH END PRESS

BOSTON, MA

Copyright © 1984 Brett Silverstein

Library of Congress Cataloging in Publication Data
Silverstein, Brett.
    Fed up!
    1. Food. 2. Diet—United States. 3. Food industry and trade—United States.
4. Nutritionally induced diseases—United States. I. Title.
TX353.S497   1984   641   84-50940
ISBN 0-89608-224-5
ISBN 0-89608-223-7 (pbk.)
Second printing
Cover design and illustrations by Ray Barnes
Typeset and produced by South End Press
Printed in the USA

SOUTH END PRESS
116 St. Botolph St
Boston MA 02115

Dedication

This book is dedicated to three organizations, the Institute for Food and Development Policy, the Center for Science in the Public Interest, and the Ralph Nader organizations, whose research and activities around the issues of food and hunger provided me not only with valuable information, but also inspiration. To the members of the Social Psychology Program at the State University of New York at Stony Brook who helped me to ask the right questions. And to my parents, Rose and Arthur, who gave me a sense of humor, the willingness to fight to make things better, and a love of food.

Acknowledgements

I would like to thank the following people for the help they gave me in preparing this book: Eileen Kelly, Linda Korkes, Jackie Lachow, Tara Losquadro, Gina Maraio, Joe Orzechowski, Fran Reilly, Gary Schiro, Carol Stewart, Eileen Sullivan, Mario Wilkowski, and the librarians at the State University of New York at Stony Brook and Columbia University helped with the research. Jan Bresnick, Louise Gikow, Deborah Perlick, Rose Silverstein, and Arthur Silverstein provided feedback on parts of the manuscript. Jeanne Dombrowski typed some of the chapters. Cynthia Peters, Ellen Herman and the rest of the South End Press Editorial Collective edited and produced the book.

The American Food System

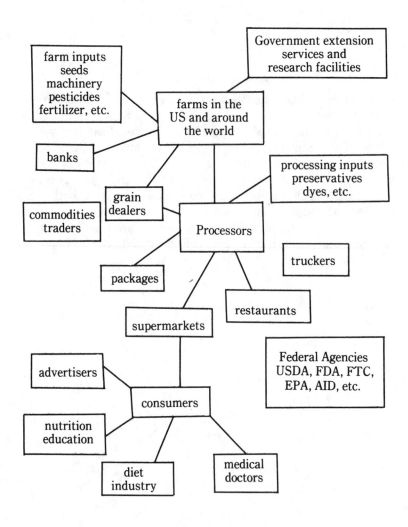

Table of Contents

Introduction

A Brazilian farmer who can no longer feed his family; a Kansas City accountant with a constant cold; a hungry child crying herself to sleep in a Harlem tenement apartment; a Dallas housewife who lives on coffee, cigarettes, and celery in order to lose weight. What do all of these people have in common? They are all being *shafted, charged, and blamed* by the American Food System.

The *shaft* assumes many forms. For Brazilian peasants it is starvation caused by forcing people off the land once used to grow their food in order to produce soybeans to be fed to American livestock. For most Americans it is tasteless and non-nutritious food, like tomatoes developed with tax dollars to be hard enough for corporate farmers to pick by machine, or like chickens which are so unhealthy that they need antibiotics because they are raised in tiny coops in chicken factories. For the American poor it is malnutrition, exemplified by government statistics showing that the diets of half of the four and five year olds in the country are deficient in niacin (see chapter 8). For perhaps 40 percent of the women in the United States it is a weight problem and constant dieting.

All of these problems and many more can be shown to result from a food production and marketing system that is designed to benefit the corporations that run it at the expense of everyone else: consumers, family farmers, small shopkeepers, taxpayers, farmworkers, women, poor people, and citizens of developing nations.

But the truth is even worse than that. In addition to starvation, poor nutrition, and obesity, the American Food System *charges* inflated food prices and the costs of unemployment. The inflation occurs, in part, because the food system is so monopolistic as to be able to overcharge consumers more than $12 billion a year (see chapter 3). High prices also result from a system that claims to be the most efficient in the world, but that uses ten calories of increasingly scarce energy for every food calorie it produces (see chapter 2), and that increases the packaging material used for fresh fruits and vegetables by 40 percent over a period of time when the per capita intake of these products has decreased by 11 percent (see chapter 4).

1

Unemployment comes about when family farmers are forced to sell their farms because they cannot compete against agribusiness, even though studies show that moderate-sized farms are more efficient than the gigantic corporate variety. The unemployment rolls are also swelled by the American farm and food industry workers who are replaced by machines or who lose their jobs when corporations decide that it is more profitable for them to exploit the cheap, politically powerless labor that is available in Third World countries ruled by "friendly" dictators. So consumers and tax-payers are forced to pay through the nose for their inadequate diet.

But the problem doesn't stop there. As if to add insult to injury, the American Food System then *blames* the economic and health problems it produces on the very people it mistreats. It claims that people in Asia, Africa, and Latin America are starving, not because their land is taken away from them to grow coffee, peanuts, or carnations for the U.S. market, but because their countries are overpopulated and they are too backward to feed themselves. It claims that many Americans suffer from poor nutrition and ill health, not because the fruits and vegetables they eat have been grown with inadequate minerals and then over-processed, or because meat-producing animals are shot up with hormones to make them grow faster, or because food is unnecessarily laden with dyes, pesticides, preservatives, and artificial colors, but because people are ignorant about the rules of good nutrition or have "picked up" poor eating habits.

The propaganda keeps coming from all directions. From the junk food commercials on daytime television to the reports of seemingly unbiased foundations that are really food industry fronts to the pro-sugar talks given by a member of a prestigious department of nutrition that received large grants from breakfast cereal manufacturers. Even the Department of Agriculture and the Food and Drug Administration contribute their share, which is not surprising once you realize that they are often staffed by former executives of food corporations who frequently return to the industry after leaving government service.

One of my goals in writing this book is to combat this propaganda. I feel that the best way to dispel the misconceptions fostered by the food industry is to make information about eating in America available to people and to allow them to draw their own conclusions about the American Food System. Another goal is to make connections: connections between starvation throughout the world, poor nutrition in America, and obesity; between racism, sexism, poverty, and poor nutrition; and between what we eat and the food industry's quest for profits. I hope that I can lift the blame for obesity, poor nutrition, and ill health from the shoulders of consumers and place it where it belongs—on the American Food System.

I wrote this book for people who are concerned about nutrition and who are trying to eat healthily; for people having trouble feeding themselves and their families because of high prices; for the rapidly growing number of people who have become concerned about the destruction of our environment; for people who suffer through diet after diet, only to regain weight and lose feelings of self-esteem and self-control; and finally, for people who want to learn about the workings of the American system. For what tells us more about a social-economic system than the way it feeds people?

Most people would probably agree that a healthy society would make good food and good health not luxuries, but rights available to everyone. In such a society, food and eating would be treated as opportunities for cultural expression and positive social inter-actions, and the production of food would be efficient, while allowing people opportunities for rewarding work and protecting the environment for future generations. The premise of this book is that while the United States could have such a society, at the present time it does not because of the control over food production and distribution exerted by giant corporations and their quest for profits. In order to understand just how this quest for profit hurts so many people, and what can be done about it, we must understand the workings of the American Food System.

The Rules That Determine Our Diet

The "American Food System" (AFS) is the term I will use to refer to the group of institutions that influence what Americans eat. The diagram on page ii shows that the AFS includes not only those institutions—farms, food processors, and supermarkets—respon-sible for producing and marketing food, but also the many institutions—government agencies, schools, banks, chemical sup-pliers, etc.—that support, supply, oversee, and otherwise affect the workings of the primary institutions. I believe that by the time you have finished reading this book, you will agree that all of the institutions that comprise the AFS play important roles in influencing our nutrition, our health, our pocketbooks, and our weight.

The AFS is large and complex, so I will wait until later chapters to detail the workings and effects of each of its component institutions. But there are a few general rules that underlie all of these specific details. Most of the decisions made by the people who have power in the AFS, and, therefore, most of the decisive influences on eating in the U.S., can be understood as attempts to follow these rules. The rules can be stated most succinctly as: "Always try to maximize 1. Profit, 2. Growth, 3. Concentration, and 4. Control."

For most Americans, the term "profit" needs little explanation. The difference between the amount of money taken in by a company for selling goods and services and the amount of money paid out by the company in order to produce and market those goods and services is profit. The total profits of the food processing industry equal about $3 billion per year.

But in our economic system, in order to maximize profit a company must strive to attain other subsidiary goals. The companies with the greatest profits, for example, are those that continue to exhibit increasing sales and the constant acquisition of new resources; in other words, growth. Growth is important because the more sales a company makes, the more profit it can make; because during periods of high inflation, everyone has to run ahead just to keep up; because as profits mount up they have to be put somewhere to earn further profits; and because if a company does not grow it will be swallowed up by another company that wants to. As a result of these pressures, American companies are like sharks that must continue to swim in order to live: they cannot remain stable. If they do not constantly move forward, they do not survive. Among the sad results of this pressure for growth, as we will see, is the need of the AFS to intentionally waste resources and to push food on people that do not need it, while others who do, go hungry. It is fair to say that the growth of the American waistline is partly due to the need for growth of the AFS.

A common mode of growth exhibited by companies is the acquisition of other companies. The end result of this process of acquisition is the concentration of resources in fewer and fewer hands. Most people do not realize the extent to which this process has already occurred. At first, small companies merged. Later, the large companies that resulted from these mergers took over small companies. Nowadays, many large companies are being taken over by even larger companies, as when R.J. Reynolds bought Del Monte, Nabisco merged with Standard Brands, and Pillsbury acquired Green Giant. So when you buy a brand name food at your local supermarket, it is probably produced by a division of a subsidiary of a giant multinational corporation. Hostess Cup Cakes, Wonder Bread, and Morton Frozen Foods are all produced by Continental Bakers, which is owned by ITT.

The resources that are concentrated in the hands of the people who run the corporate giants that result from these acquisitions are overwhelming. The $11.3 billion in sales by Cargill, a grain dealer that most Americans have probably never heard of, is larger than the gross national product of most African nations. Beatrice Foods, another corporation unknown to most Americans, has acquired over 400 companies since 1894, including Dannon yogurt, Louis Sherry ice cream, La Choy oriental foods, Tropicana fruit drinks, Eckrich Meats, and Samsonite luggage, and employs 88,000 people.

One effect of increasing growth and concentration is increasing control. Companies strive to control as many of the aspects of their business as possible. Control can mean the mechanization of farming and processing to control workers, research grants to control the food technology that is developed, lobbying and campaign contributions to control government decision making, advertising and marketing tricks to control consumer choices, and even genetic manipulation to control the biological makeup of crops. When control is in the hands of a few corporations, they are able to plan strategy, to reduce uncertainty, and to manipulate others, all of which mean greater profits.

The quest for profits sometimes leads the AFS to use cheap ingredients (see chapter 3) or unsanitary procedures (chapter 10) when producing food. The quest for growth sometimes leads the AFS to push junk food on children (chapter 6) or fattening food on overweight adults (chapter 9). The quest for concentration sometimes leads the AFS to promote giant farms that use unhealthy amounts of pesticide (chapter 1) or to promote processed rather than fresh food because processing allows nationwide sales and brand-name advertising (chapter 3). The quest for control sometimes leads the AFS to support dictators in underdeveloped countries who, in providing cheap land and labor to food corporations, often exacerbate the hunger of their own people (chapter 11) or to fight labelling laws that would help consumers to better understand what they are purchasing (chapter 4).

The problem is not simply one of evil executives and greedy corporations. These exist, but they are more a result of a misfunctioning system than its cause. The way the rules of our food system are set up, corporate executives cannot afford to be nice guys. If, for example, the board of directors of Food Inc. (a fictional company), that produces a fictional food called "flammus," were to decide to improve the nutritional state of Americans by using higher quality, more expensive raw "flammus" in its product, or if, upon discovering that children are eating more "flammus" than is good for them, it were to stop advertising on children's television shows, the profit, growth, concentration, and control (P-G-C-C) of Food Inc. might decrease. When the decrease became large enough, either the board of directors would be replaced by angry stockholders, or Food Inc. would be swallowed up by some other corporation whose lack of public spirit allowed it to continue the more profitable, but less healthy, practices. So, if the board members of Food Inc. want to maintain their positions, they have no choice but to try to maximize P-G-C-C. Corporations that place the public welfare above their own quest for P-G-C-C soon cease to exist. As long as the American Food System remains in its present form, the rules will have to be followed, and the American diet will, in large part, be determined by the corporate quest for profit, growth, concentration, and control.

To understand just how this quest produces eating problems and then blames them on us, and what we might do to solve these problems, we have to uncover some of the astonishing facts and crazy stories about the different parts of the system. Chapter 1 demonstrates how recent changes in farming have reduced the quality and variety of the American diet, taken away the livelihoods of many farmers, and wreaked havoc on small towns and on the environment. Chapter 2 shows how technology has been misused, resulting in crops that are less tasty, jobs that are less rewarding, and food production that is more expensive. Chapter 3 details how the factory processing of food adds needless chemicals to our diet and allows the food manufacturers to overcharge us. Chapter 4 points out how supermarket managers eager to sell their most profitable items use many tricks to confuse shoppers and to influence our food purchases. Chapter 5 provides evidence that while convenience foods may sometimes be useful, they are often expensive, non-nutritious, and not even very convenient. Chapter 6 makes the case that food advertising is meant to manipulate consumers, not to inform us, and that it promotes poor nutrition, obesity, higher prices, and crazy attitudes toward food, particularly among children. Chapter 7 describes the ignorance of most Americans, including doctors, nurses, and teachers, about nutrition and shows how the food industry propaganda is often used to teach nutrition in schools. Chapter 8 discusses some of the links that have been drawn between nutrition and health and the reasons that U.S. health care tends to ignore nutrition and to focus on drugs and surgery. Chapter 9 shows that weight and eating disorders ranging from obesity to chronic dieting and dissatisfaction with our bodies are not simply individual ailments that should induce guilt and embarrassment, but are social problems that must be dealt with by making changes in the food system, particularly in the way women are treated. Chapter 10 argues that while government decisions sometimes improve the American diet, all too often these decisions are subverted by pressure from the food industry. Chapter 11 attempts to prove that the chronic hunger experienced by millions of people in Third World nations is not due to ignorance or overpopulation but to corporate profit-seeking actions that are similar to those that produce the many problems described in earlier chapters. Finally, Chapter 12 draws some general conclusions about what must be done to solve these problems.

Most Americans are unaware of the extent of these problems, which are getting worse. The first step in doing something to improve the situation is learning just what is going on, and there is no better topic with which to begin this process than where our food begins—the American farm.

The Chicken Story

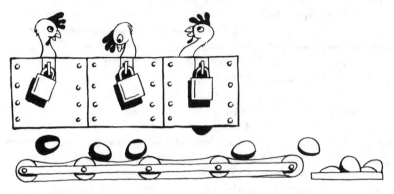

If you grew up singing "Old MacDonald" you probably think that a chicken farmer awakens each day to the crowing of the rooster and walks outside to be greeted by a barnyard full of chickens, clucking and scratching and pecking the earth in search of bugs, worms, and fallen kernels of corn. This image is romantic, but unrealistic. In the U.S., food is a business; business means profits; and profits mean factories, machinery, and chemicals. As a result of research done on the breeding of broiler chickens, a mature four-pound bird can now be produced in about half the time, using half the grain, that it took twenty years ago.[1] The research was promoted by large corporations involved in food processing and feed production, like Pillsbury and Ralston-Purina. These companies took control of poultry-growing by signing chicken farmers to contracts that specified how many chickens were to be raised, under what conditions, and at what prices. It reads like a great success story for the American Food System. In their quest for increased profits, the corporations streamlined the production process and everybody benefitted.

Well, maybe not everybody. In order to keep their farms, chicken farmers need capital from the corporations, virtually forcing them to sign the contracts. Often they must deal with a corporation that has a monopoly over the poultry business in a particular locale or with a small number of corporations offering very similar contracts. Either the farmer signs the contract, thus agreeing to all of the conditions specified by the corporation, or goes out of business. Having little bargaining power, the farmer gets

9

little return. The USDA estimated that in 1964 poultry farmers received one cent an hour for their labor.[2]

Today, most chickens are grown in what can only be called chicken and egg factories. They are kept indoors and fed from automatic conveyor belts. They deposit their manure on other belts which drop it into huge pits. Their growth is stimulated by manipulating artificial light to simulate longer days. They are plucked by machines. They are kept warm in winter and cool in summer by electrically driven heaters and fans.

It's expensive to raise chickens this way, so the chicken output must be large to make it profitable. Flock size in the typical egg factory is between 20,000 and 80,000 birds. In order to accommodate such vast numbers, chickens are crowded together or cooped up in tiny cages stacked on top of one another. The stress produced by crowding and unhealthy living conditions (dust, bacteria, ammonia from the manure pits, lack of sunlight or mobility) leads to cannibalism and disease. Tranquilizers are sometimes used to reduce the cannibalism. More often the problem is solved by machines that de-beak the birds.

Disease reduces the lifespan of modern laying hens from a possible fifteen to twenty years to an average of about one and a half years. To combat the disease and to promote fast growth, antibiotics, sulfa drugs, and sometimes arsenic are added to chicken feed. Other feed additives include colorants like xanthophyll or beta-carotene, which create yellow skins and egg yolks. Fungicides decrease feed spoilage. Pesticides are sometimes added which pass through the birds' digestive tracts and remain in the manure, to reduce the fly population in the manure pits. The slaughtered chickens are bathed in tetracycline and ascorbic acid to increase their shelf life. They are also immersed in water and chlorine to reduce bacterial growth, a practice that has been banned in the European Common Market countries. Although modern techniques allow less water absorption during cleaning than was previously possible, poultry processors often see to it that they reach the legal limit in absorption in order to increase the weight of each bird.

Along with water, consumers get lots of fat. As a result of breeding for fast-growing birds, chickens contain more fat than they did twenty years ago. According to the agricultural handbook put out by the USDA, the amount of raw fat in chickens tripled between 1960 and 1979.[3] According to the book *Animal Factories* by Jim Mason and Peter Singer,[4] factory eggs are smaller and have less yolk than eggs produced a decade ago. They are also paler, more watery, and lower in two B vitamins, B12 and folic acid, than eggs from barnyard hens.

Farming

One-seventh of the meat and poultry for sale in supermarkets contains pesticides in amounts that are above the legal limit.[1] This sad situation exists because the food industry has come to dominate farming and livestock raising and has instituted methods of growing food that are based on the mass production techniques used in its factories. As a result, even fresh food is less healthy than it once was.

In the industrial mode of production for private profit, single products are manufactured in giant mechanized factories with the help of chemicals whenever natural processes "break down" or proceed too slowly for big profits. This description applies equally to a plastics plant, a bread factory, a tomato farm, or a beef feedlot because plastic, bread, tomatoes, and beef are all simply products from the point of view of industrial corporations.

If, according to the trade journal *Farmer and Stockbreeder,* "the modern layer [hen] is, after all, only a very efficient converting machine, changing the raw material—foodstuffs—into the finished product—the egg—less, of course, maintenance requirements"[2] then it follows that livestock raising, and by extension the growing of any food, is just one branch of industry. As a result, livestock are increasingly being raised in gigantic mechanized feedlots that some have called "animal factories."

Tremendous resources are invested in the U.S. livestock industry. Each year American livestock consume about ten times as much grain as is consumed by the total U.S. population.[3] In the United States, almost half of the plant protein fed to animals is in the form of grain, much of which could be eaten by people. This is wasteful because eating grain is more efficient than feeding it to animals that turn some of it into meat and the rest into hooves and bones and the energy for heat and movement. It takes about seven times the amount of fuel and sixteen times the amount of labor to provide one gram of animal protein as it does to provide one gram of plant protein.[4] Thus, whereas less than half of the American diet comes from animals, 90 percent of the energy used for growing food is used for animals, which adds to the cost of food.[5]

A steer raised in a feedlot on grain has more fat than a grass-fed steer raised on the range, so grain-fed animals grow rapidly and produce tender meat. Grain feeding provides the animal industry with faster-growing, more profitable animals, and it provides the American consumer with steak that is tender but increasingly expensive, bacon that is so fatty it disappears in the skillet, and a diet that promotes obesity and heart disease.

As a result of the financial and health problems caused by eating lots of meat many people are trying to replace some of the meat in their diet with grain and vegetable dishes. Perhaps the major obstacle preventing even more people from doing so is ignorance about how to easily prepare tasty, healthy, cheap dishes based on grains or beans. In the last few years a number of books have been published that present arguments for eating less meat and that give recipes for non-meat dishes. Some of these books are listed in the Appendix.

The inefficiency of animal production increases when animals are shipped from the farm to feedlots. Farm animals can eat home-grown fodder and bits of grain that fall to the ground during harvesting; feedlot animals must eat high-energy grain that has to be brought from the farms. Farm pigs can regulate their own temperature using soil, shade, and mother's body; feedlot pigs have to be heated and cooled with electric devices. Chicken manure can be used as fertilizer on farms; the manure of feedlot chickens is just a health hazard, polluting the water and increasing sewage costs for local communities. In fact, animals supply about two tons of manure each year and half of that is from feedlots.[6] According to one estimate, if the manure from feedlots was used for fertilizer it would provide almost as much energy as that which now comes from expensive synthetic fertilizer.[7]

But using natural fertilizer would be a poor way of expressing gratitude to the chemical industry that does so much to affect our food supply. Over 1,000 drugs are approved by the FDA for livestock and poultry.[8] These include Hog Krave, used to artificially stimulate the appetite of pigs in order to fatten them in a hurry, prostaglandins, used to induce labor contractions in pregnant animals in order to give farmers more control over the timing of births, other sex hormones—estradiol, progesterone, and until it was prohibited in 1979 after many years of fighting, DES—used to stimulate rapid growth in cattle, and millions of pounds a year of antibiotics, used to promote rapid growth and to fight disease in sickly feedlot animals.

One result of this massive use of antibiotics is that bacteria that are frequently exposed to the antibiotics develop immunity to them through a process of evolution. Those bacteria that have a natural immunity to a widely used antibiotic are the ones most likely to survive the treatment of animals with that antibiotic. When these bacteria reproduce they pass on the immunity. As a result, after repeated contacts with an antibiotic many of the surviving bacteria are immune. Many bacterial strains attack both humans and animals so promoting immunity in the bacteria that prey on livestock may produce health hazards for people. Unfortunately, there appears to be no way to prove that using antibiotics on animals increases human susceptibility to disease, so the livestock industry, which profits from the uninhibited use of antibiotics, has succeeded in defeating most efforts to regulate the use of these drugs on animals.

Besides being inefficient and unhealthy, animal factories are inhumane. The animals are crowded together unable to move. They may get no sunlight, their manure builds up to unhealthy levels, and they are bred for fast growth, overtaxing their bone structure and producing deformities. For example:

1. Light-colored, tender veal comes from calves that are tied by their necks to prevent movement, fed milk replacer containing no iron in order to produce that anemic light flesh, and confined in stalls with no straw or bedding because the starved animals would eat them and thus ingest iron.

2. In order to produce pigs as fast as possible, farmers must artificially inseminate breeding sows at exactly the time that they are in heat. To discover when that time is they keep some males around. But animals being what they are, this might lead to fooling around, so some farmers have the penises of the male pigs removed or surgically rerouted to exit their bodies at the flank. These latter animals are referred to as "sidewinders."

The Industrial Farm

The industrial model of growing food affects crops as well as animals. Classic farming methods such as crop rotation, the use of manure as fertilizer, and the planting of alternate rows with different crops produce healthy food while protecting the land. They were developed over centuries to meet the needs of farmers who eat some of what they grow and who want to pass on their way of life to future generations. These methods make sense to farmers who value self-sufficiency and have a long term stake in their land. They do not make sense within a corporate system that treats farming as an industry and food as a commodity, that can move to new land whenever it has to, and that profits from methods of growing food that necessitate the purchase of expensive chemicals and machinery by farmers.

The problems begin before the crops are planted, with the seeds on which our food supply is based. For thousands of years the seeds for one season's crop came from the crop of the previous season. But corporate farmers wanted the higher profits that come from faster-growing crops. So, in the same way that scientists, at the prompting of the food industry, developed fast-growing chickens, they applied genetic research to develop hybrid seeds (the results of cross-breeding different varieties of a crop) that grow faster and produce higher yields. Like fast-growing chickens which are fatty and prone to disease, however, the fast-growing seeds have many disadvantages. The switch to the new seeds affects the variety in our diet, the security of our food supply, and the quality of our food.

As more farmers use the new seeds the variety of crops available to the consumer decreases. How many different kinds of apples have you tried? You've probably tasted Delicious, Mac-Intosh, Granny Smith, Rome Beauty, and perhaps three or four other varieties. But have you tasted the Pippin, Spitzenburg, Gravenstein, Northern Spy, Baldwin, Astrokahn, or any other of the 8,000 varieties of apples catalogued by the USDA at the end of the 19th century? One hundred ninety-seven varieties of corn exist, but according to the National Academy of Sciences almost three-quarters of U.S. corn acreage is planted in only six different varieties,[10] half of all American wheat comes from nine varieties of seed, two-thirds of sweet potatoes come from one variety of seed, three-quarters of potatoes come from four varieties, almost all peas come from two varieties, and all of the millet in North America comes from three varieties of seed.

This lack of variety is more than a boring inconvenience; it is a danger. As the Irish learned during the 19th century potato famine, a food supply that lacks variety is vulnerable. Organisms that are dangerous to plants, like certain bugs, weeds, funguses, viruses, and bacteria, usually attack one plant variety and spare others. When hundreds of varieties are planted, the destructive organisms may kill the crops of a few fields but the resistant varieties survive. But when thousands of farmers plant just a few varieties, destruction can run rampant. Aggravating the problem, hybrid seeds tend to have less resistance to pests and disease than do ordinary seeds. The National Academy of Sciences warns that "most [U.S.] crops are impressively uniform genetically and impressively vulnerable."[11] In 1970, the fungus Helminthosporium maydis destroyed one-seventh of the U.S. corn crop. The disaster cost the nation $1 billion and ruined some farmers but it did not change corporate farming methods.[12]

The new seeds may also produce lower quality food. David Perelman, in his book *Farming for Profit in a Hungry World*, reports that Indian corn is richer in every essential mineral than modern, commercially grown corn.[13] By 1956, some samples of hybrid corn had a protein content of about half that of traditional non-hybrid corn in 1911. Since that time, the increased use of fertilizer has produced some increase in overall protein content, but may also have produced a decrease in the levels of two components of protein that are necessary for the proper utilization of protein in the body. Hybrid corn may also be low in boron, cobalt, and sulphur.

The problem is certainly not confined to corn. The Peruvian-Bolivian potato contains almost twice as much protein as American potatoes. According to the USDA, some American wheat is so low in protein that it is unfit for milling. In a sane food system this nutrient loss would be cause for alarm, but if you ran a corporation that gets paid for each can of corn sold, would you promote the use of seeds that produce more nutritious corn or seeds that produce faster-growing corn?

The new seeds have other advantages for the food industry because they are hybrids produced by cross-breeding which, like mules, cannot reproduce themselves. This means that farmers can no longer provide some of their own seeds; they are more dependent than they used to be on companies that produce seeds. This state of affairs is perfect for corporations seeking to increase profits and their control over the food supply. Sensing new opportunities, large U.S. conglomerates have begun to acquire seed companies. Purex owns Ferry Morse, Sandoz owns Northrup King, and ITT owns Burpee.[14] A number of other corporations, most of them in the oil, chemical, or drug industries, have recently purchased seed companies as well.

Exacerbating this dangerous trend is the recent passage of laws that allow seeds to be patented. Never before could private enterprise own all of the rights to a life form. Four corporations already control two-thirds of the hybrid corn planted in the United

States.[15] Four corporations also hold over three-quarters of the patents on beans.[16]

Chemical Farming

In order to flourish, the hybrid seeds need lots of water, fertilizer, and pesticide. The oil, drug, and chemical corporations that own seed companies are unlikely to develop seeds that need few applications of the chemicals they produce. In the words of two representatives of the chemical industry:

> We look at the progressive farmer of today as an associated businessman in the chemical industry...After all, these men [sic] are producing proteins, fats, celluloses, carbohydrates—all of which are processed chemicals. The goal of this chemical plant operator is not to grow a crop of lettuce, a herd of steers, etc. but to maximize his [sic] return on investment.[17]

Modern agriculture is based on massive applications of synthetic nitrogen, phosphorous, and potassium fertilizers. Whereas the soil used to be the major source of plant nutrients, it now serves as a base to support plants doused with artificial "food." The use of fertilizers has replaced crop rotation. Before synthetic chemical fertilizer, planting a field of the same crop year after year depleted the soil of its nutrients and eventually led to failed crops. Now, major nutrients are supplied by the fertilizer.

Unfortunately, synthetic fertilizer does not contain all of the nutrients that are found in the soil. Trace minerals like zinc and selenium that occur in tiny amounts in the soil and in the human body are crucial to health. Without crop rotation soil may become entirely depleted of these trace minerals. So will we. Nobody knows how far this process has already progressed on farms.

The environmental effects of heavy fertilizer use are not known. In some areas where extensive applications of nitrogen fertilizer (the most common type) are combined with heavy irrigation, the nitrogen-nitrate concentration of the ground water supply has been found to be dangerously high, threatening the population with nitrate poisoning and perhaps cancer.[18]

The amount of fertilizer used on American farms has increased over sixteenfold since 1935[19]—just about the time that small family farms began to disappear and farm size began to increase. This is not a coincidence. The large farms fostered by the food industry are the ones most likely to use chemical farming methods. In a study of wheat farms in Montana, the USDA found that large farms used 50 percent more fertilizer per acre than small and medium-sized farms.[20]

Pesticides

The other important chemicals used on modern farms are pesticides. Approximately one billion pounds of pesticides are used in the United States each year to kill insects, weeds, and fungi.[21] These pesticides also kill other organisms. In the Southwestern United States in the 1960s pesticides caused the death of a massive number of birds.[22] In an incident in California in 1974, over 2,000 ducks were killed by pesticides. Over one-quarter of the bees kept in the San Joaquin Valley of California in 1972 were killed by a pesticide, which also contaminated 35,000 tons of alfalfa. And the brown pelican, the Louisiana state bird, has been just about eliminated by insecticides.

Human beings, particularly farm workers, are also poisoned by pesticides. The California Department of Public Health found that 90 percent of farm workers report some symptoms of pesticide poisoning.[23] In a Florida study, one out of ten poisoning deaths were found to be due to pesticides.[24] These dangerous chemicals are ingested regularly by American consumers. Many of the 143 chemicals known to leave residues in meat and poultry are pesticides.[25] Over one-third of these chemicals are suspected of causing, or have been proven to cause cancer or birth defects or mutations, and many of the chemicals have never even been tested.

Most of the chemicals that leave residues in food are not regularly monitored. For the pesticides that are monitored, the levels that are legally allowed in inspected food are set individually for each food. These levels do not take into account that someone may eat several contaminated foods simultaneously. Furthermore, as the long-term effects of chronic pesticide ingestion are unknown, they are ignored in setting legal limits. Even with these low standards the General Accounting Office found that inspection for pesticides was lax. When contaminated food is found, punishments are very minor—perhaps a warning on the first offense and small fines thereafter.

Due to all of these problems a great deal of pesticide is being ingested by people that eat the typical American diet. The World Health Organization has calculated Acceptable Daily Intake levels for various pesticides, which are believed to be low enough to protect adults against a dangerous buildup of these chemicals. In 1976 the U.S. Environmental Protection Agency measured the amount of pesticides ingested daily in breast milk by nursing babies. Comparing these two sets of figures, the Environmental Defense Fund found that for the pesticide DDE the average intake by American babies in mother's milk is over twice as high as the safe level for adults, and for the pesticide dieldrin, the average breast feeding American baby ingests over nine times the amount of pesticide defined as safe.[26]

The problem is not limited to this country either. The amount of pesticides exported from the United States almost doubled over the last fifteen years.[27] One-quarter of these pesticide exports are products that are banned, heavily restricted, or have never been registered here. When tests show that a pesticide is too unhealthy to use, the chemical companies do not cease producing it, they dump it on unsuspecting countries. When Hooker Chemical Company (of Love Canal fame) voluntarily withdrew the registration of the pesticide BHC after tests on mice showed that even in tiny concentrations it causes tumors and premature births and kills fetuses, the company stated that it would continue to produce BHC and to export it overseas.[28]

As a result of practices such as these, the World Health Organization estimates that one Third World person is poisoned by pesticides every minute.[29] But the story gets even worse. The people being poisoned do not benefit from the food on which the pesticides are sprayed. It has been estimated that over half of the pesticides used in underdeveloped countries are applied to crops that are exported to Europe, Japan, and the United States.[30] So not only are people overseas subject to pesticide poisoning, but American consumers ingest, in imported food, pesticides that have been banned here because they produce health problems. The FDA found that one-tenth of our imported food contains illegal levels of pesticides and the General Accounting Office found that almost half of all imported green coffee beans contain at least some residue of pesticides banned in the United States.[31]

Perhaps the most ironic part of the story is that overspraying pesticides actually makes pest control more difficult. Like bacteria frequently exposed to antibiotics, pest species that come into frequent contact with pesticides eventually develop resistance to the chemicals. Between 1962, when Rachel Carson wrote *Silent Spring*, and 1971, the number of resistant pest species almost doubled.[32]

Also, some plants and insects live by killing pest species. Often the pesticides destroy these predators as well as the intended pests. After the spraying, the pests may re-invade; because of the lack of predators the destruction of crops can be worse than ever. Sometimes a previously unimportant species can become a pest after its predators are killed and it is allowed to multiply unchecked. The spidermite became one of California's major insect pests in this way. In 1976, the California Department of Food and Agriculture found that of the twenty-five most serious pests in the state (those that cause at least one million dollars of damage) three-quarters were resistant to at least one pesticide, and the problems caused by all but one were either created or aggravated by pesticides.[33] Between 1942 and 1978, insecticide use in the United States increased over tenfold while the rate of crop loss to insects doubled.[34]

So why do American farmers use so much pesticide? First, because the planting of the same crop, over large areas, year after year, using hybrid seed, leaves crops very vulnerable to pests. Second, although a combination of biological, chemical, and other farming methods has been found to be very effective in combating pests, and costs much less than the completely chemical approach, the chemical companies that control the pest control industry block the usage of these methods.

They accomplish this by supporting research to develop new chemicals but not to perfect and apply nonchemical means of pest control. In the words of a spokesperson for the National Agricultural Chemical Association, "There really is not much biological control in industry research, they would research themselves right out of the market."[35]

You might think that the institutions that invest large sums in agriculture would be able to fight the wasteful use of pesticides. But, according to a representative of the Bank of America, which invests heavily in agriculture, "We're not really concerned about the effective use of pesticides; why should we be? We have billions invested in the chemical industry."[36]

Who Controls Agriculture?

Between 1935 and 1974 the size of the average farm in the United States tripled, while 2,000 farms went out of business each week.[37] A recent study by the California Institute of Rural Studies found that in California (which has the largest dollar value of farm produce of any state) fewer than 4 percent of all the farms control more than half of the crop land.[38]

The shift to giant farm agribusiness is usually justified in terms of efficiency. Agribusiness spokespeople point to the difficulty of using modern farming techniques on small farms and claim that we must have large farms if we want to feed everyone. They fail to mention that very large farms are also inefficient. Giant farms need many levels of management; decisions are often made by absentee owners; resources are not used as carefully on large farms as on smaller farms; workers do not work as hard when they are not directly benefitting from the work. As a result, study after study finds that moderate-sized farms are as efficient or more efficient than small or large farms.[39]

Giant farms are profitable because the owners pay lower interest rates on loans and lower prices for supplies than do the owners of moderate-sized or small farms. According to an extensive report on farm size and efficiency: "...since farms are motivated by total profit rather than by [maximum efficiency], we should expect farm operations to gravitate toward sizes well beyond the most efficient size."[40] According to Jim Hightower, recently elected Texas State Agricultural Commissioner, three-quarters of California's vegetables in 1972 were produced on farms that were much larger than the optimum size.[41]

As family farmers have been losing control of their land, the corporations have been gaining control. For example, by 1980 the Tenneco Corporation, originally involved in oil and chemicals, controlled at least one-tenth of strawberry and table grape production in the United States and almost three-quarters of almond and date production.[42] Tenneco owned or leased over two million acres of land. Tenneco's control over the food we eat was increased by its ownership of storage facilities and distributors. Tenneco's subsidiaries include the Packaging Corporation of America, J.I. Case Machinery (the third largest farm machinery company in the United States), Tenneco Chemical Company, which produces, among other things, flavoring for processed foods and raw materials for fertilizer, and the Newport News Shipbuilding Company, which produces ships to transport food. (Other conglomerates that have been "farmers" at one time or another include American Cyanamid, Bunge, Del Monte, Goodyear, Libby, Minute Maid, Swift, United Fruit, and Standard Oil.)

The most important recent change to occur in the organization of farming has been the development of contract farming. Food corporations have realized that farming is too risky. In a typical contract arrangement, the corporation gets the benefits of controlling the farming without taking the risk by providing the farmer with the capital needed to buy supplies and agreeing to purchase from the farmer a fixed amount of a specified variety of produce at a prearranged price. While contracts may differ, the corporation usually has the right to specify the conditions under which the produce is to be grown. This may include the seeds to be planted, the type and amounts of fertilizers and pesticides to be applied, the drugs to be given to animals, and the equipment to be used.

Farmers have little or nothing to say. If the corporation wants them to use expensive equipment, they'd better do so or risk losing the contract. Banks may only give credit or lease some of their massive landholdings to farmers who agree to use the modern industrial methods that the industry favors. If farmers don't agree, they go out of business. Corporations like Del Monte or Green Giant often have the right to decide which produce is acceptable for purchase and which is not. The farmers can then sell their rejected asparagus, for example, to Del Monte for a fraction of the regular price, or they can live on asparagus for the next year. Some contracts even state that the corporations "are not responsible for errors in judgment," so if the choice of seed or fertilizer produces a bad crop, the farmer pays, not the corporation.

Industrial Farming and the Environment

These changes will have long-lasting effects on the environment as farming methods suited for producing rapid profit are not suited for careful conservation of resources. The boards of directors of agribusiness corporations think in terms of one year, sometimes five to ten years, but not in terms of generations. A manager who went to one of these boards with a farming project in which profits would be moderate but in which the environment would be protected would be laughed at, if not fired. As a result, American cropland is being wasted and destroyed.

The U.S. has always been a great place for growing food. The fertile soil and temperate climate combine to make one-fifth of the land arable (i.e. suitable for farming).[43] This is a much higher proportion than in other areas of the world, four times the proportion of farmland in Africa or South America. In fact, the United States has one-seventh of the good farmland in the world, and there is three times as much farmland per person here as there is in the rest of the world.

But, while American farmers use the abundant farmland that allows the United States to be a major exporter of food more efficiently than they once did, they continue to be less efficient than the farmers of many other nations.[44] In 1977, twenty-six countries produced more wheat per acre than the United States, with some, such as France and the Netherlands, growing more than twice as much per acre. The U.S. did much better in corn production, but Australia, Canada, Italy, and Switzerland did still better. In oat production, the U.S. was tied for twentieth place with Hungary.

At the same time we are frittering away the good land with which we started. During the last 200 years, at least one-third of American topsoil has been lost to erosion.[45] Industrial farming methods were responsible for much of this erosion. In Missouri, annual soil erosion rates averaged seven times as much per acre on land planted continuously with one crop compared to land on which traditional crop rotation methods were used.[46] The gigantic tractors that are used on the large farms crush the soil under their weight and need so much room to maneuver that farmers have to tear out trees and bushes that protect the land from wind erosion. In some irrigated areas, groundwater is being pumped up so fast that the water table is dropping and the land is sinking. As a result of environmental problems such as these, American farms lose billions of dollars worth of soil nutrients each year.[47]

In addition to the physical environment, corporate farming damages the social, economic, and cultural environment of a community. Perhaps the best evidence for this is a series of landmark studies in which sociologist Walter Goldschmidt compared two California communities of similar size, population, and agricultural output, but differing in the type of farms that surround them.[48] Dinuba was a town surrounded by small, family farms, whereas Arvin was surrounded by large, "modern" farms. Goldschmidt found that compared to Arvin, Dinuba had twice the number of separate business establishments, 61 percent more retail trade, three times the amount of expenditures on household supplies and building equipment, 20 percent more people supported for each dollar of agricultural produce, a higher average standard of living, and more parks, schools, civic organizations, newspapers, paved streets, sewage and garbage disposal, and churches. The population around Arvin consisted of a few, relatively well-to-do farm owners and many low-paid migrant agricultural workers, neither of which identified with the community. You don't have to be a mystic to believe that the methods a society uses to grow its food and the way it treats animals and the land will have major repercussions not only on the health of that society but on its entire way of life.

The Tomato Story

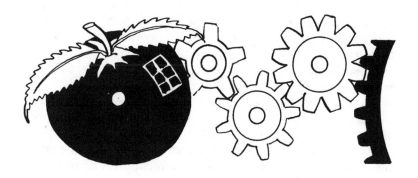

If you are old enough to compare the taste of tomatoes available in supermarkets nowadays with those available fifteen years ago, or if you have recently eaten home-grown tomatoes, you have experienced some of the effects of technology on food quality. To understand the causes of the downfall of the American tomato, we must look at recent changes in tomato farming technology.

Until recently, many tomatoes were grown on small farms located throughout the country. But the owners of supermarket chains prefer the ease of dealing with a few large packers who can supply tons of tomatoes throughout the year rather than with many small farms on a seasonal basis. Because of this and other factors, tomato farming became centralized on giant farms in California, Florida and (for processing tomatoes) Ohio. Many consumers began to eat tomatoes that had travelled a thousand miles.

The next development occurred when farmworkers began to unionize. It is quite difficult to organize workers who are constantly migrating, but once organized, farmworkers have a lot of power. Imagine threatening the owners of giant farms with a strike just when thousands of acres of tomatoes are ripe and ready to be picked. The farm owners and the processors who hold the contracts for the produce could not stand this loss of control. They responded by promoting the development of machinery that could replace the farmworkers.

For this plan to work, the owners needed the help of professionals: engineers to develop the machines, biologists to breed new varieties of tomatoes that would make the usage of machinery economical, chemists to develop chemicals that would control the ripening process and others that would control pests.

The industry offered researchers at state agricultural colleges, particularly Davis in California and some midwestern state universities, money to be used to develop the new technologies. This was a wise use of funds for agribusiness corporations because they had only to supply relatively small amounts of tax-deductible funds in order to gain access to scientists, laboratories, and equipment that were supported by tax dollars. One study estimated that over a fifteen year period, Purdue, Michigan State University, and Ohio State University received about $300,000 from agribusiness corporations for research on the mechanization of tomato harvesting, while the public supplied about $750,000 for that research.[1]

Of course, the people who run the universities were happy to oblige. Why shouldn't they be? Many of them profited from the research. William K. Coblentz, chair of the University of California Board of Regents in 1978, was also the managing owner of ASA Farms, owner of a million dollar parcel of tomato cropland in Yolo County, California.[2] Edward W. Carter, another member of the Board of Regents, owned $78,000 worth of stock in Del Monte.

What were the effects of these changes? First, small farmers were pushed out of business. A harvesting machine, which costs $40,000 whether it is used on thirty acres or 300 acres, is much more profitable for large farmers. In 1963, before tomato harvesters were used, California had over 4,000 tomato farms, averaging thirty-two acres of tomatoes each. By 1973 about 600 farms were left, averaging over ten times as much tomato acreage.[3]

Second, farmworkers lost their jobs or were forced to work for lower wages. In 1976, the electric-eye, mechanized tomato sorter displaced 5,000 California farmworkers. Those who found jobs had to take a twenty-five cent an hour wage cut.[4] In some cases the machinery was more expensive to use than was farm labor. Given that for each sixty-cent, one-pound can of tomatoes, only two and a half cents goes to the grower,[5] reducing the cost of farm labor would not seem to be the most important priority for consumers. One California tomato grower admitted that mechanized sorting is more expensive than hand sorting, but added "one of the big advantages of these machines is you can keep the people you want and get rid of the trouble makers."[6]

As a result, the price of food has not even been reduced by the technology. Between 1964 and 1978, the price of tomatoes increased more than the price of retail food and almost three times as much as the price of strawberries, which are harvested with very little mechanization.[7]

Finally, the quality of tomatoes has suffered as a result of the new technologies. In order to insure that tomatoes would not rot by the time they reached distant supermarkets, and in order to ripen most of their tomatoes simultaneously, growers began to pick the tomatoes before they ripened and then artificially ripen them using ethylene gas. In order to prevent the destruction of the tomatoes in transit and to allow the tomatoes to be picked by machine (even though many fresh tomatoes are still hand-picked), new varieties of tomatoes, tougher than the old varieties, were developed. The result is the tasteless, hard tomatoes on sale at our supermarkets.

The destruction of the tomato is highlighted by the story told by Thomas Whiteside, who visited Florida to research an article on the new tomatoes. In order to demonstrate the resourcefulness of the tomato industry, one industry representative tossed the new MH-1 tomato into the air and let it fall to the ground. The skin remained unbroken. Whiteside sent the figures on how far that tomato had dropped to a friend in Detroit, who calculated that it had survived a fall impact of 13.4 miles per hour; over two and a half times the U.S. government standards for auto bumpers.[8]

Technology

If the Wizard of Oz were made today, Dorothy, upon spotting the tornado, would run home to find her Uncle Henry and Auntie Em rushing around trying to protect their tractor, reaper, harvester, and automatic grain dryer. Science, technology, and mechanization have swept the modern farm and food industry. Spokespeople for the industry brag about their technological efficiency but people have recently begun to realize that, in and of itself, technology is neither good nor bad. What matters is who controls it, what it's used for, and who pays for it. Nowhere is this clearer than in the mechanization of farming.

The most obvious effect of farm mechanization has been the major change in the way Americans earn their livings. In 1850, almost two-thirds of the U.S. labor force were farmers; nowadays, less than one out of thirty laborers work on farms.[1] Mechanization forced many small farmers, who could not afford the expensive machinery that was developed for large-scale profitability, to become hired farm workers. Many other farmers and farm workers displaced by machinery had to move to the cities to find jobs in factories.

Some of this displacement was intentional. In 1970, when the United Farm Workers went on strike against the lettuce growers, the growers donated $13,500 to the University of California to develop a mechanical lettuce picker. In the words of Roger Garret, the engineer who developed the picker, "The machine won't strike, it will work when [the growers] want it to work."[2] The food industry brags about the efficiency demonstrated by eliminating so many "surplus" farmers and claims that the average farmer used to be able to feed only three people and now he or she can feed forty.[3] As usual, this boast of efficiency is misleading, for while some labor was replaced by machines, much of it was not so much replaced as transformed.

In the nineteenth century, most of the work done to supply food to Americans was done on the farm. Nowadays, much work is put into food after it leaves the farm. According to the Bureau of the Census, in 1978 about two million people were employed in food processing, over two million worked in retail food stores, over four million worked in restaurants, soda fountains and other enterprises, and about a million worked in the trucking and warehousing of food, and the production of farm and garden machinery.[4] These figures do not include people who manufactured, distributed, or sold cans, boxes, labels, seeds, refrigerators, or microwave ovens.

Some of the new jobs created by mechanization were in high-paying, technical professions and required much skill. But the changes made by the food industry in the twentieth century fragmented the work of farming and reduced the amount of skill needed on most jobs. People who might have been farmers in the past, with a wide range of skills and knowledge about crops and climate, are now hired farm workers who walk behind harvesting machines sorting fruit. Most butchers have been replaced by assembly lines in meatpacking plants where workers continually repeat just one step of the butchering process. Many grocers, who used to have to understand produce, marketing, and people, have been replaced by teenagers stacking and stamping cans. Checkout clerks, who at least had to know prices and be able to work cash registers, have recently been turned into human robots who simply pass packages by computerized sensors. Chefs, even in many "fancy" restaurants, now thaw out frozen entrees, and waiters and waitresses are being replaced by fast food workers who simply hand out packages. In order to maintain maximum control over the work process and to pay the lowest wages possible, the food industry has transformed interesting jobs requiring skill into repetitive, mindless tasks. Whereas apprentices used to work for years learning a trade, most jobs nowadays can be learned in days, weeks, or perhaps a month.

What effect does all of this have on the consumer? First of all, most consumers are workers too and, as Harry Braverman showed in his brilliant book *Labor and Monopoly Capital*,[5] the forces that have robbed workers in the food industry of their skill and their independence have had the same effect on most other occupations. Increased mechanization and scientific management of work go hand-in-hand with industrial farming and processing and their bad effects on our diet, our culture, and our environment. The chicken and tomato stories, recounted at the beginning of the first three chapters of this book demonstrate what can happen to food quality when technology is used solely to increase profits. Most of the costs for developing these technologies are paid for by taxpayers who support state agricultural colleges. The machines also cost taxpayers in other ways; increased unemployment produced by automation forces many people onto the welfare rolls. Finally, food production requires energy. If that energy is not supplied by human beings, it must come from other sources. That brings us to perhaps the most inefficient and costly aspect of our food system.

Energy

Where once farmers and horses worked the land, today we have automatic harvesters and tractors. Where once animals on farms consumed grass, today we have animals in air conditioned feedlots eating grain. Where once rotating crops and spreading manure provided nutrients to the soil, today we have petroleum-based artificial fertilizers. Where once careful farming practices combated insects and weeds, today we have pesticides, also made from petroleum. Where once grain dried in the fields, today we have propane-fueled grain driers. Where once fresh food provided sustenance, today we have highly-processed food packaged in plastic, yet another petroleum derivative. Where once food was consumed near its point of production, today we have giant, centralized farms and factories necessitating much transport and storage between the farm and the table.

All of these changes increase the use of nonrenewable fossil fuel. For example, in 1970, we got 25 percent less energy from corn for every calorie that went into growing the corn than we did in 1945.[6] In a classic article, John and Carol Steinhart estimated that, not counting the energy used in trips to the store or in hauling garbage, the food system accounted for more than one-tenth of total American energy usage in 1970.[7] They concluded that "in 'primitive' cultures five to fifty calories were obtained for each calorie of energy invested...In sharp contrast, industrialized food systems require five to ten calories of fuel to obtain one food calorie." So the "efficient" American food industry wastes energy in the midst of possible scarcity and saves labor in the midst of unemployment.

If American methods of food production were used to feed the world, even if petroleum were used only to produce food, the world's total petroleum reserves would last a mere twenty-nine years.[8] Yet these methods are being instituted in many nations throughout the world. Some are even touted as being the answer to the problems of hunger in the underdeveloped countries. But a closer look at the most important of these, "The Green Revolution," will demonstrate that technology designed to produce profit seldom helps people.

The Green Revolution (GR) refers to the development of the hybrid seeds discussed in the first chapter, along with the development and implementation of the technology needed to use the seeds. The research upon which the GR is based was sponsored by industrial interests, particularly the Rockefeller Foundation, in what has been touted as a selfless use of American know-how to solve the food problems of underdeveloped nations. Norman Borlaug, the chief researcher, received a Nobel Prize for his role in the Green Revolution.

But, looking beneath the surface, we find that, like modern American farming methods, while the Green Revolution technology saves time, land, and labor, it does so at a cost. The innovation of the GR was not so much breeding faster-growing crops. The Chinese had been doing that since the Sung Dynasty in the eleventh century. The key to the GR was the development of crops that respond well to irrigation and to artificial fertilizers. The GR seeds were bred to thrive, but only under excellent conditions—few pests, much water, and lots of fertilizer. They are more sensitive to disruption of these conditions than are traditional varieties. As in the U.S., the new seeds must be repurchased each year. So, to use the GR seeds a farmer needs a great deal of money, usually in the form of credit, controlled irrigation, which often means a tubewell, and much technical support.

As a result, the landless peasant, the tenant farmer, and the small landowner have a great deal of difficulty using the GR technology. They cannot get credit so they must borrow at exorbitant rates from the large landowners who can. They do not have the time, the education, or the connections to get help from the government unless it is made easily available, which is usually not the case. They often cannot afford to risk their livelihoods by borrowing heavily to finance GR technology. One bad year and they would lose their land.

With technology, land becomes more valuable, increasing the power of landlords and creating attractive investment opportunities for wealthy city-dwellers. As the profits to be made from growing food for the urban and overseas markets increase, tenants are thrown off the land and small landowners are swallowed up. Many studies find that when GR technology is introduced into an area the size of the average farm, the amount of land controlled by the wealthiest people, the amount of food exported to wealthier nations, and the number of landless laborers increase, while the number of farms, the number of fulltime jobs, and the salaries of the laborers often decrease. In other words, the rich get richer and the poor get poorer.

In the words of former Secretary of Agriculture Clifford Hardin:

> The impact of these new GR grains—which double, triple, and even quadruple yield—goes beyond crop yields. They alter basic farm practices; they increase the demand for fertilizer, pesticides, tillage machinery, pumps, engines, wells, and for such things as transistor radios and motorbikes by farmers able for the first time to buy them with profits from increased production. They can become powerful engines of change in national economies in the less powerful underdeveloped countries.[9]

Translated, this means that the new technology produces a need for farm equipment manufactured in the United States, creates a middle class to buy U.S. luxury goods, displaces farm labor in order to provide workers for new industries, and provides new sources of crops for export by agribusiness firms. It also increases the concentration of landownership throughout much of the world as well as the control exerted by landowners, credit institutions, and corporate sources of farm equipment over the economies of many nations and over the lives of many millions of people. Meanwhile, peasants who had been feeding themselves, albeit at a minimum level, can no longer afford to do so. Production of food increases along with the number of hungry people.

In some cases, technology has benefitted the majority of the people. A study of two similar villages found that in Sahimal, Pakistan, where land was very inequitably distributed and access to credit for tubewells was given primarily to large landowners, the GR technology increased the inequity.[10] However, in Comilla, Bangladesh, where land was more equally distributed and village cooperatives formed to make use of the technology, most of the village benefitted. Other nations, that have more equitable distribution of land, such as Cuba, Taiwan, Japan, and China, have also been able to implement technology to good effect.

Clearly technology in itself is not the problem. Science and technology can aid us in providing more and better food for everyone and can save workers from unnecessarily arduous labor. Small scale technology can easily complement, rather than replace, human labor. We have reached a point where careful implementation of technologies that are already available, and others that could easily be developed given the state of modern science, can be immensely beneficial to most people.

In order to make proper use of technology, two points must be kept in mind. First, there is no such thing as a free lunch. That is to say, the land, energy sources, people, plants, atmosphere, and animals that comprise our food system are interrelated; a change in any part will produce changes in the others. As a result, the use of technology to improve just one aspect of the production of food will have effects on the other aspects of the process. Faster-growing chickens come at the expense of increased drug usage and higher fat content. Automated baking of bread adds chemicals and reduces nutritional content. Tomatoes bred for shipping and machine-harvesting are hard and tasteless. All technological processes use energy and affect the number and quality of available jobs. If we are careful we can decide to use technology only when the benefits it brings are greater than the costs it produces.

Who Controls the Technology?

But, in most decisions about whether or not to implement a particular technology the costs and benefits are not given equal weight because, in general, the benefits of the technology (e.g. profit) go to people other than those who pay the costs. When that happens, the people benefitting will try to increase the use of that technology. Similarly, when some people have something to lose from a technology that benefits the majority—such as cars that last for decades or cheap, effective, nonchemical means of pest control—they will not try to develop that technology and may even find ways to subvert it. As a result, the effects of technology will very much depend on who controls its development. In the United States the control is in the hands of agribusiness corporations that have great influence over the scientists that develop food technology and do research on food and nutrition problems. One study found that for each tax-deductible donation of one dollar, the agribusiness corporations can influence state agricultural colleges to commit four dollars' worth of resources, in the form of laboratories, equipment, and salaries, to projects chosen by the corporations.[11] According to the Auditor General of the California state legislature, this research even extends to brand name products.[12]

But industry money buys even more than technology that "helps the big get bigger," in the words of former Secretary of Agriculture Bob Bergland.[13] It also buys experts who issue pro-industry statements to the media and who testify in front of government committees. Often these experts appear to be unbiased. For example, the Council for Agricultural Science and Technology (CAST), which was organized at Iowa State University "to advance the understanding and use of agricultural science and technology in the public interest,"[14] sounds scientifically neutral, doesn't it? The truth is that most of the funding for CAST comes from dues from chemical companies such as Dow, Monsanto, and Hoffman-La Roche, and from such organizations as the National Corn Growers Association and the Florida Fruit and Vegetable Association, as well as from grants from Ralston-Purina, General Mills, and other agribusiness corporations. CAST press releases and reports to government agencies, however, mention only the scientific organizations affiliated with the council. The reports issued by CAST have discouraged actions against pesticides, nitrates, school breakfast cakes, and animal antibiotics. Seven scientists in the task force that researched the antibiotics report resigned in protest charging that the report was slanted in favor of antibiotics.

Other unbiased-sounding supporters of the food industry include the Nutrition Foundation, the National Commission on Egg Nutrition (which, according to the FTC, sounds like "an impartial, independent, quasi-governmental health commission when in fact it is an association of persons engaged in the egg industry,"[15] the Institute of Food Technology Expert Panel on Food Safety and Nutrition, and the American Council on Science and Health (ACSH), which gets funding from industries other than the food industry but which includes on its board of directors many members who have received support from food corporations.[16]

Among the directors of ACSH is a person whose credentials and institutional affiliation would seem to make him a highly credible expert on food and nutrition: Professor Frederick J. Stare of the Harvard Department of Nutrition. Doctor Stare's views, publicized through interviews, lectures, and columns, might make you feel a little less worried about the effects of the food industry on the American diet. He has been quoted as claiming that "most people could healthily double their sugar intake daily" and that there is "[no] reason for concern about food chemicals."[17] He has testified in Congress and in FDA hearings on behalf of Carnation Milk, the Sugar Association, Kellogg, and Nabisco. The catch is that the Harvard Department of Nutrition receives large sums from numerous food and chemical corporations, including Carnation, the Sugar Association, Kellogg, Nabisco (do these names sound familiar?), Coca Cola, Monsanto, Nestle, Pepsico, and Oscar Mayer.[18] In the three years after he told Congress that "breakfast cereals are good foods," Stare's department received $200,000 from Kellogg, Nabisco, and their related foundations.

To make matters worse, committees appointed specifically to advise the government also exhibit conflict of interest. The Food and Nutrition Board associated with the quasi-governmental National Academy of Sciences' National Research Council is extremely influential regarding food policy. In 1980, the Food and Nutrition Board issued a report that concluded that "healthy people need not worry about fat and cholesterol."[19] The report ignored many studies to the contrary and overlooked weaknesses in the studies it did cite, perhaps, in part, because six of the fifteen members of the task force that produced the report were employees of, consultants to, or received funding from organizations such as the American Egg Board, the National Livestock and Meat Board, and the National Dairy Council. No epidemiologists or any scientists known to be worried about cholesterol were included in the task force.

Thus, we live in a world where science and technology can help us to live easier, more enjoyable lives and eat a better diet. But when technology is instituted to promote an industry's profit rather than to improve the lives of farmers and consumers, when control of the technology is not in the hands of the public, when technology replaces human beings who do not have the opportunity for other meaningful work or forces people to become merely adjuncts to machinery, when the application of technology ignores the social, cultural, political, and economic contexts in which it is used, when concern for minimizing the use of labor or land is at the expense of other concerns such as saving energy and providing healthful food—then the public's needs will not be met. In other words, when technology is used by the few to increase profit, the result will be the unemployment, boring jobs, giant farms, high prices, energy shortages, environmental decay, cultural disruption, fatty chickens, spongy bread, and hard tomatoes that we have been experiencing recently, not to mention the chronic hunger and mass starvation that exist in many underdeveloped nations today. Unfortunately, science, which could be so helpful to people, has become mainly a servant of private profit. As you are about to learn, this is one of the reasons that we eat so much processed food nowadays.

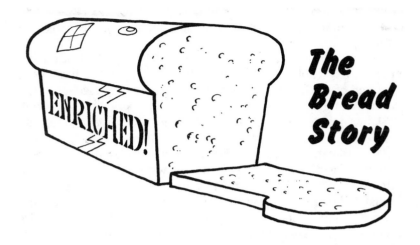

The Bread Story

Bread has been baked for thousands of years, but in the twentieth century, the baking process in the United States has undergone vast changes. The germ of the wheat (the part of the wheat kernel that develops into the wheat plant) contains oil, so bread made from whole wheat goes rancid after a while. The germ also includes much of the nutrient content of the wheat, so it attracts bugs and rodents. The solution of the baking industry to the rancidity and pest problems was mechanical milling, which eliminates the germ, and with it the oil and the nutrients. (Well, at least the bugs don't get them!) It also eliminates the bran (outer layer) of the wheat, which contains most of the fiber.

But mechanical milling and baking was not good enough. Chemical techniques were adopted to make the process faster and more profitable. In order to speedily whiten the flour and to make it easier to bake with, bleaching and maturing agents were employed. Until 1946, nitrogen trichloride was used for this purpose. However, when tests showed that nitrogen trichloride produces symptoms of hysteria in animals, industry bakers shifted to other bleaching and maturing agents, like benzoyl peroxide[1] which, according to the Clearasil package, is the strongest acne medicine available without a prescription!

The baking industry uses many other chemicals to make the job of mechanically baking bread easier and faster. A typical loaf of commercial white bread contains calcium propionate, to inhibit mold growth; benzoyl peroxide, chlorine, or chlorine dioxide, to bleach the flour; magnesium chloride and magnesium carbonate, to prevent the caking of the dough and to increase its flow; potassium bromate, to speed up the fermentation process; mono- and diglyce-rides, to retard staling; as well as salt, sugar, and other ingredients.[2]

Many of the vitamins and minerals in bread are lost during processing.[3] Whole wheat flour contains at least two to three times as much of the following nutrients as refined (i.e. mechanically-milled) white flour: thiamine (vitamin B1), riboflavin (B2), niacin (B3), pyridoxine (B6), biotin and folic acid (other B vitamins), calcium, magnesium, copper, zinc, and phosphorous.

In order to deal with this depletion of nutrients, the bread industry fortifies refined white bread with extra vitamins and minerals and labels the bread "enriched." Unfortunately, the industry does not mention that of the sixteen or so nutrients lost during refining from flour used to make bread, only four are replaced. The levels of these four nutrients (thiamine, riboflavin, niacin, and iron) are then out of balance with the other nutrients that have been processed out of the bread and may not be efficiently utilized by our bodies. Natural vitamins that are lost are replaced by cheaper synthetic versions. Some nutritionists believe that synthetic nutrients are as good as natural ones, but others stress that we are not yet knowledgeable enough about nutrition to insure that every important aspect of a natural product is being reproduced in the synthetic version.

Anyone who has eaten homemade bread or fresh bread from a bakery knows that bread is not processed to improve its taste. Nutritionist Jean Mayer has stated that in his native France, the soft, white, tasteless substance that so many Americans eat would not even be called bread.

Processing

Can you imagine filling a five-pound bucket with the contents of a chemical laboratory and then swallowing the mixture? Well, you don't have to imagine it because that is just about what you do over the course of a year when you eat the typical American diet.[1] Americans today eat more processed food unnecessarily laden with chemicals than ever before.

In 1930, the average American ate almost twice as many fresh vegetables as processed vegetables.[2] Now he or she eats many more processed vegetables than fresh. In 1940, the average American bought three pounds of frozen foods, while in 1976 he or she bought almost ninety pounds. Food processing has become a multibillion dollar industry that relies on complex machinery and thousands of chemical additives.

Sometimes the chemicals are added to food in a real attempt to improve it. More often, additives are used so that food can be processed by machine, canned or frozen, dehydrated or drowned in liquid, shipped across the country, and stored for months, while retaining some small resemblance to what some of us remember as fresh food.

For example, to prevent oil from separating out of such products as peanut butter or artificial whipped cream, the processors use emulsifiers. To thicken watery mixtures like soft drinks, ice cream, or baby foods, they use stabilizers. To add taste to many processed foods, they use artificial flavors. To trap metal particles that enter machine-processed or canned food, they use sequestrants. To maintain moisture levels in candies and marshmallows, they use humectants. Acidulants and antioxidants are used to preserve food, and firming agents and conditioners are used to make processing quicker, easier, and more profitable.

Salt and sugar are used not only to put some taste and cheap bulk into processed foods but also to allow storage for long periods. Both of these substances appear in products ranging from soup and gravy to breakfast cereals and pancake mixes. Unfortunately, while the processors may benefit from the frequent use of salt and sugar, we do not. According to the USDA and the Senate Select Committee on Nutrition and Human Needs, the intake by most Americans of both salt and sugar is much too high.[3]

Not every chemical in food is bad. Even some of the synthetic additives with long names, like ascorbyl palmitate, a vitamin C derivative used to prevent rancidity, play useful roles, and may do more good than harm. But many of them are harmful. Some allow manufacturers to use shoddy methods of preparation or inferior ingredients. In the words of an advertisement placed by a producer of additives in *Food Engineering*, a magazine read by food processors, "Textaid puts uniform, rich, pulpy texture where it's needed to restore natural food appearance lost in heat or processing."[4] While some manufacturers of ice cream produce high-quality products without any additives, others must add stabilizers, like gelatin or carboxymethylcellulose, so that they can use cheap ingredients without ending up with a lumpy, watery product.

Other additives do harm by replacing or destroying more nutritious ingredients. Processed peanut butter contains up to 10 percent mono- and diglycerides to keep the oil from separating. These chemicals take the place of the extra peanuts that are used in natural peanut butter, which contains 100 percent peanuts.

Some additives do more direct physical harm. Caffeine has been shown to cause birth defects in animals, is believed by some researchers to be related to breast lumps in women, and is known to affect the human nervous system. Yet it is added to cola drinks to replace the caffeine that naturally occurs in cola, which is lost during processing. A can of cola may contain half as much or more caffeine than a cup of coffee. No wonder it is often difficult to get the kids to sleep.

A number of additives have been banned, for health reasons, by the FDA and the USDA. Polyoxyethylene-8-stearate, a synthetic emulsifier used in baked goods, was found to cause bladder stones and tumors.[5] Cobalt salts, a synthetic stabilizer used in beer, was found to have toxic effects on the heart. Nordihydroguaiaretic acid (NDGA), an antioxidant derived from a desert plant, was found to cause kidney damage. Safrole, a flavoring derived from sassafras that was used in root beer, was found to cause liver cancer.

Unfortunately, these additives were used in food for many years before being banned, and the results are not in on many other additives that are being used today. For example, modified food starch is natural starch that has been chemically treated to prevent it from precipitating or clumping and to make it less fragile. It is used to thicken many foods, including some baby foods, replacing more nutritious ingredients and possibly affecting digestion in infants. The United Nations FAO/WHO (Food and Agricultural Organization/World Health Organization) expert Committee on Food Additives reported in 1970 that modified food starch was being used without being adequately tested.[6] Carrageenan, another substance that we don't know enough about, is used to thicken soft drinks, ice cream, and jellies, to gell puddings, and to prolong the shelf life of infant formula.[7] Millions of babies, therefore, have ingested chemicals that may be dangerous.

Even when processors add nutrients to food, they do not do us any favors. Capitalizing on the trend toward more consciousness about nutrition, the food industry has taken to fortifying some products, particularly cereals and baked goods, with vitamins and minerals. But this practice can lead to some pretty ridiculous situations. Do you want your kids eating enriched "Twinkies" for breakfast? That's what they are doing when they eat the cream-filled, sugar-laden cakes made by ITT and Tasty Bakers for school breakfasts. Kellogg's Frosted Rice Cereal contained 25 percent of the U.S. recommended daily allowance of iron until it was discovered that the ground particles of iron that were being used to fortify the cereal were not being evenly distributed; consumers were able to move flakes of the cereal with magnets.[8]

Flavors

Most food additives are used as flavorings or flavor enhancers to replace, or mask the absence of more expensive natural products, and to improve the taste of machine-processed food. The flavor enhancers (e.g. maltol and ethyl maltol, disodium guanylate and disodium inosinate, and monosodium glutamte) allow processors to skimp on meat in soups, gravies, and stews. MSG (monosodium glutamate) has been found to cause brain and retinal damage in infant mice, but processors fought for years to keep it in baby food, even though it was used to improve the taste for mothers who bought the food, not for the babies who ate it. Babies are less sensitive to some tastes than are adults. Finally, the industry, faced with the overwhelming evidence presented by food activists, admitted defeat and took the MSG out of baby food.

Two-thirds of the additives used in the United States are natural or synthetic flavorings.[9] Most flavors have not been tested for safety, based on the logic that they are used in small amounts and may occur naturally. Some of the natural flavors that have been tested, however, have had to be banned because they cause such problems as liver cancer (safrole) or intestinal tumors (oil of calamus).[10]

Imitation flavorings are each made up of from 10 to 100 ingredients (chosen from about 2,000 possibilities) by expert flavorists, who use chemical methods and sensitive noses and tongues to analyze the components of natural flavors. They pride themselves on being able to reproduce thousands of flavors ranging from strawberry and chocolate to chicken and human breast milk. They can even reproduce the taste of canned tomato paste which includes the tinny taste of the can.

At first, these imitation flavors were used, almost apologetically, to supplement natural flavors. Recently the industry has become bolder, sometimes completely replacing natural flavors with artificial flavors and bragging that they are going nature one better. Flavoring companies advertise in industry magazines that their imitation coconut flavor "tastes more like coconuts than coconuts" and that "sophisticated dairy flavors aren't born. They're made."[11]

It is impossible to tell whether company representatives are lying or have finally lost all of their ability to differentiate what is real from what is not. In either case, the quest of the food industry for profits ("Spectra chesse flavors deliver substantial savings...Now when he says 'Cheese' you can say 'Profits'"[12]) is leading us to a situation described by one food flavorist:

> In twenty years, I'll bet that only 5 percent of the people will have tasted fresh strawberry, so whether we like it or not, we people in the flavor industry will really be defining what the next generation thinks is strawberry. And the same goes for a lot of other foods that will soon be out of the average consumer's reach.[13]

In fact, we may have already arrived. One company recently ran an ad for "our new apple flavor...Tart and tangy, it's just right for today's trend in nostalgic flavors."[14]

In addition to taste, factory processing robs food of important nutrients.[15] Fruits lose half of their pantothenic acid (a B vitamin) during canning, vegetables lose a third to a half of their vitamin B6 during freezing, and many meats lose most of both of these vitamins during processing. Spinach loses four-fifths of its manganese, beans lose three-fifths of their zinc, and carrots lose almost three-quarters of their cobalt during canning. When rice is polished it loses many of these minerals, which are necessary for good health.

Processing also upsets the necessary balance between nutrients in food. In order to function properly the human body must maintain a balance between sodium and potassium. But the processing of canned peas lowers the potassium content of raw peas by two-thirds at the same time that it increases the sodium content fourteen times.[16]

Why So Much Processing?

Industry spokespeople would have us believe that all of these problems are minor compared to the advantages we derive from processing. In an article in the prestigious *Journal of the American Dietetic Association,* F.M. Clydesdale wrote that "To achieve year-round food availability, we must accept loss in nutritional value" that comes from processing.[17] There is some truth to this statement. Foods have growing seasons. Without processing, we would be unable to eat these foods wherever and whenever they are not in season. But, in most parts of this country there is still a large variety of unprocessed or slightly processed (e.g. plucked chickens) food available any time of the year. When you cannot get grapefruit, you can get cantaloupe. When you cannot get summer squash, you can get winter squash.

Fresh food in season tastes delicious. Have we really gained much if we trade taste and nutritional value for year-round availability? What's so great about non-nutritious, tasteless food that is available all of the time?

Industry representatives also use exaggeration to make light of the problems resulting from food processing. The same article that advises us to accept nutritional loss, justifies the use of potentially dangerous chemicals in food by asserting that "...there is no such thing as an unqualifiedly safe drug or safe food. Even spinach will harm you if you eat too much of it." Again there is some truth to this statement, but what it is really saying is that since eating 20,000 peanuts will kill you, you may as well not worry about the carcinogens (cancer causing chemicals) put into your food. "No additives means no condiments, no salt, no pepper, no sugar—rather a monotonous outlook," writes Mr. Clydesdale. In other words, people who complain about the sodium erthyorbate in liverwurst or the monosodium glutamate in gravy are really trying to deprive us of mustard for our meat and pepper for our eggs.

When the processed food industry gets tired of defending itself, it attacks. In a recent annual report, International Flavors and Fragrances, a producer of food additives, implied that synthetic foods may be preferable to natural foods, which really consist of "a wild mixture of substances created by plants and organisms for completely different non-food purposes—their survival and reproduction."[18] Beware of apples, they were created for making baby trees, not for pies.

As you can see, the arguments of the food industry, especially if they are made by experts, must be taken with a grain of salt (you see, we do need additives). But why does the industry mislead us? Because although processing may not always benefit us, it certainly benefits the food industry.

To see how this works, let's go to the supermarket to buy a pound of potatoes. When we head to the produce aisle for a sack of raw potatoes, we discover that a pound of potatoes costs sixteen cents (1980 prices). But over in the canned food aisle, that same pound of potatoes, in the form of slightly processed Del Monte canned potatoes, costs thirty-three cents. In frozen foods, a slightly more processed pound of Oreida Tater Tots costs forty-two cents, and Safeway frozen french fries cost fifty-one cents a pound. In convenience foods, a pound of Betty Crocker Potato Buds costs $1.05 a pound, and a pound of Proctor and Gamble Pringles Potato Chips in the snack section costs $1.91.

The more processed the food, the more we pay. Part of the price increase is due to the cost of labor and materials, but a good deal of it is not. The eleven-fold increase in price between a pound of raw potatoes and a pound of potatoes in the form of potato chips is hardly due to the cost of salt, oil, sugar, packaging, and labor.

The first rule of food processing is: if you perform a service or add an ingredient that costs two cents, you can raise that price four or six cents. In the words of Tenneco's California Almond Orchards, "...adding almonds to your products costs only a fraction of a cent. But almonds add a lot of flavor, texture and glamor to your product. So you can charge a few cents more."[19] Wheaties cereal is the same product as Total, but Total has a few cents' worth of synthetic vitamins added. Wheaties costs ninety-six cents a pound and Total costs $1.60 a pound.[20] (Dr. Michael Jacobson, of the Center for Science in the Public Interest, advises people who buy Total to replace it with Wheaties and some vitamin pills.)

Much of the increase in food prices that has occurred in the last thirty years has gone into the pockets of food processors. Even when you pay the same for a serving of factory-processed food as you do for a serving of homemade food, it is usually because the processed variety uses cheaper, lower-quality ingredients. After all, the food industry is hardly interested in doing extra work for nothing, so it is not hard to figure out why food companies want you to eat canned, frozen, or prepared food. If you ran a food corporation and knew that when you added a cheap chemical or fooled around with the food in some other way you could get back more than your costs, would you produce and push fresh food or the highly processed variety? Why, you might even come to share the sentiments described by Adolph S. Clausi, of General Foods, a member of the Food Engineering Hall of Fame, who said, "In the packaged food industry the word 'commodity' means a food product that is relatively easy to produce and pack [i.e. an unprocessed food], a not very distinctive product with a low profit margin. In fact, in my business, 'commodity' is sort of a bad word."[21] Aren't you glad to know that the people in charge of your food supply think that "fresh" is a dirty word?

Besides being more profitable, food manufactured with lots of chemicals tends to vary little from month to month and can be stored easily, freeing processors from worries about bad weather, labor disputes, and farm prices. In the words of the Arthur D. Little Company report to the food industry, "The further a product's identity moves from a specific raw material—that is, the more processing steps involved—the less vulnerable is its producer."[22] So Monsanto can offer processors interested in purchasing its synthetic chocolate flavor, "The true taste of chocolate made entirely without chocolate (and without the vagaries of today's cocoa market)."[23]

Processing also allows the most powerful food companies to get bigger because it makes for easier labeling and advertising and because processed food can be shipped across the country, allowing for national rather than local markets. And processed food is manufactured in expensive factories, making it more difficult to start new companies, so processing serves to decrease competition in the food industry.

What About Competition?

Many Americans have grown up thinking that in this country competition is a hallmark of our economic system and that this competition forces businesses to come up with new ideas and to produce the best products at the lowest prices. But nowadays, in many industries, a few giant companies can avoid competition by controlling most of the sales and by taking over smaller companies. General Foods, one of the largest of these conglomerates in the food industry, provides a good example of this process.

The General Foods company was born in 1891 when Charles William Post was a patient at the Battle Creek Sanitarium, a health spa run by the Kelloggs. While he was there he was impressed by a coffee substitute, subsequently called "Postum." Soon the Postum Company began to market cereals like Grape Nuts and Post Toasties. Then the mergers began. In 1925 the company acquired the Jello Company. In 1926 it acquired Ingleheart Brothers, makers of Swans Down cake flour, and the Minute Tapioca Company. In 1927 came Franklin Baker, maker of coconut, Walter Baker, maker of chocolate, and Log Cabin, the syrup company. Meanwhile, Clarence Birdseye had returned from the Arctic, where he had seen Eskimos preserving meat by freezing it. He invented a commercial method for freezing foods and, in 1924, he founded the General Foods Company.

In 1929, the Postum Cereal Company bought General Foods and took over its name. Later the company acquired Gaines dog food (1943), Kool Aid (1953), Good Seasons salad dressing (1954), and Open Pit barbecue sauces (1960), among many other companies in the United States and overseas. Today, General Foods produces all of the aforementioned products as well as coffee, including Maxwell House, Yuban, Sanka, Brim, Max Pax, Maxim, and General Foods International Coffees. (General Foods and Proctor and Gamble now sell almost two-thirds of the ground coffee in the country.[24] General Foods and Nestle sell over three-quarters of the instant coffee.) The company also sells many pet foods, including Gravy Train, Prime, Top Choice, and Cycle, as well as many breakfast drinks, among them Orange Plus, Start, and Tang. Also marketed by General Foods are Shake 'n Bake, Pop Rocks, Cool Whip, Stovetop stuffing, Hollywood chewing gum, Burger Chef fast foods, and other products in many countries, including France, Spain, Sweden, Brazil, Japan, and Australia.

As a result of this type of acquisition process, small food manufacturers are disappearing and large processors have come to dominate the industry. By 1974, the fifty largest food companies representing a tiny fraction of the total number of food companies, accounted for almost 90 percent of all food processing profits.[25]

The next time that you visit the supermarket, notice how many of the products in each aisle are made by just a few companies. Are most of the soups made by Campbell? Are most of the vegetables canned by Green Giant or Del Monte (recently taken over by the R.J. Reynolds Tobacco Company)? Are most of the ketchups made by Heinz or by Hunt? In 1978 nine-tenths of the ketchup bought by Americans was produced by three companies.[26] Three companies also made just about all of the frosting sold in the United States that year. In fact, according to the USDA, control by a few companies is the rule rather than the exception in the manufacturing industries.[27]

With decreased competition comes increased profits and increased prices. According to studies done by the Federal Trade Commission (FTC), in the most highly concentrated food industries (those that are controlled by a few companies), the rate of profit is much higher than in the food industries that are not so concentrated.[28] When concentration in an industry is high, the controlling companies tend to avoid price competition. Instead, according to the USDA, "competition in concentrated...industries mainly occurs in terms of product variations, package design, advertising, and promotion. Costs for these are passed on to the consumers in the form of high prices."[29]

This is not a small problem. According to one study, in 1978, as a result of concentration in the food manufacturing industry, American consumers were overcharged by $12 to $14 billion.[30] To put this sum into perspective, it means that every time that we spend $20 on food, we are overcharged more than $1 due to concentration among food processors.

The giant corporations would have us believe that concentration is good, or at least inevitable, because it results when the most innovative and efficient companies keep growing. In rare moments of honesty, however, corporate executives have admitted that giant corporations are not as innovative as smaller businesses. In the words of Anthony J.F. O'Reilly, the chief executive officer of the H.J. Heinz Company, "...the best way to get into new product development is to take over some other guy's idea by buying the company."[31]

Larger corporations do not create, they acquire. They grow by using their financial power to take over smaller companies. That kind of growth produces no new ideas, no new products, and no new jobs. One of the weaknesses of "supply-side" economic theory is inherent in this expansion. Supply-side claims that the way to promote productivity in the United States is to help corporations acquire as much wealth as possible, which they will supposedly use for productive investment. The problem is that when corporations get their hands on money they do not use it for new production. They use it to buy other corporations. Since money is thus spent without creating anything new, these acquisitions fuel inflation while increasing neither production nor employment.

For the last fifty years or so, food corporations have increasingly moved into industries—both food and nonfood—other than those in which they began.[32] General Mills bought Parker Brothers (appropriately, the manufacturer of the game Monopoly); Swift and Company beefpackers (now called Esmark) bought Playtex bras; Pepsico bought Wilson sporting goods; Ralston-Purina bought the St. Louis Blues hockey team; Borden bought Krylon spray paints; and Nabisco bought Serutan laxatives. Each of these corporations also owns many other nonfood companies. This move toward diversification allows the corporation to avoid great losses should business slow down in one industry, and to put smaller companies out of business by temporarily reducing prices for one product while maintaining profits in other areas. It does not lead to the production and sale of better food.

There is no reason to be surprised that companies that produce soft drinks or bacon also produce basketballs or panty-hose, for the food industry is like any other industry. It relies on industrial methods of marketing and advertising. Unfortunately for our taste-buds, our pocketbooks, and our health, it also relies on industrial methods of production. As a result, you would be better off if you ate fresh food whenever possible. You cannot always do so, but, by referring to the books on additives listed in the appendix, you will at least be able to avoid the most dangerous chemicals put into your food. But the food industry does not even inform us of all of the additives that it puts in food, which is only one of the marketing tricks discussed in the next chapter.

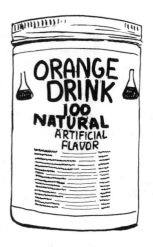

The Health and Natural Food Story

The food industry uses product descriptions like "pure," "organic," and "natural" on its labels to mislead us. Not surprisingly, the industry that makes much of its profit from processing food is hardly in the vanguard of advocating unprocessed food. The industry issues reams of trade journal articles and public relations pamphlets about the harmlessness of food additives and the advantages of using pesticides, preservatives, dyes, etc. But, while the industry is powerful, it is not omnipotent. It has been unable to completely outflank the advocates of health-and-nutrition-consciousness. Sales of Pringle's potato chips dropped drastically after an ad campaign by a competitor pointed out all of the additives that they contained.

In recent years, the industry has worked out an "if you can't beat 'em, join 'em" strategy that exploits health consciousness to sell supposedly healthful products. From Flintstone vitamins, containing more sucrose (one of the many words for sugar that appear on food labels) than any other ingredient, to Quaker 100% Natural Cereal, with six grams of sugar per ounce, the industry sells commercialized, inferior versions of healthful products.

Perhaps most indicative of this trend is the industry's use of the word "natural." To most of us "natural" probably means "containing nothing artificial," but not to the food industry. Pace Natural Strawberry-Flavored Yogurt has natural strawberry flavor, but the yogurt contains a preservative and artificial color. Kraft Cracker Barrel Natural Cheddar Cheese contains potassium sorbate and artificial orange color. "Natural orange flavor" Tang contains sugar, citric acid, maltodextrin, calcium phosphate, potassium citrate, artificial flavor, celluose and xantham gum, artificial color, and BHA. The "natural" on the label is used to signify that a single ingredient in the food is not artificial. Tang contains a little bit of real orange flavor so it can be labelled "natural orange flavor" and still contain artificial flavor.

One of the newest marketing tricks is based on the growing awareness of shoppers that whole grain products are much healthier than products made from refined flour, leading people to switch to whole wheat bread. In response, some bakers are making their white bread look more like whole wheat by darkening it with caramel colors and changing the name to wheat bread. White bread was always made from wheat, but from refined wheat, not from whole wheat. If the first ingredient listed on the label is not whole wheat flour, it is not whole wheat bread. The change in color and name are clearly designed to confuse shoppers.

Marketing

The Case of the Supermarket Swindle

As she deposited her son Billy in the front seat and her shopping bags in the back seat of the '77 Chevy on that unseasonably warm November day, Sally Shopper had no reason to suspect that anything unusual had just happened. Her morning coffee had taken the last drop of milk in the house and the bread supply was low, so, after picking up Billy, she had stopped at the supermarket on the way back from the library. She bought a loaf of bread, a gallon of milk, a box of cereal that Billy wanted, a few cans of vegetables and a few cans of soup, some frozen dinners, six (or was it eight?) apples, a package of cheddar cheese, a box of mint candies, a few items that appeared to be on sale, a few others that caught her eye, and a magazine that she noticed while waiting in line at the checkout counter. With her parcels in a cart and Billy by her side, she returned to her car, not knowing that she had just been victimized in the Crime of the Century. She had been manipulated, misled, overcharged, and confused. She had made uninformed purchases which contained unnecessary chemicals, had paid an unwarranted sum and remained unaware of the process.

You too are frequently victimized in this recurring crime. The evidence is there if you know where to look and the perpetrators have left a trail of clues that can be followed, but only by a cagey supermarket detective. The trail starts with the money you give to supermarket owners.

Between 1958 and 1976 the food retailers' share of your food dollar increased by 20 percent, in part due to increasing concentration within the retail food industry.[1] Small grocery stores are disappearing and supermarket chains now sell more than half of the food bought by Americans. The four largest retail food companies in each metropolitan area studied in 1972 averaged over half of the sales for that area.[2]

When a few chains control sales in your neighborhood, profits go up and, in the words of a report to the Joint Economic Committee of Congress, "...the higher observed profits are due at least in part to the higher prices that chains are able to charge in less competitively structured markets."[3] The result is a nationwide overcharge in food bills due to monopoly in the retail food industry in 1974 conservatively estimated at 625 million dollars.[4]

When members of the industry are accused of profiteering they protest their innocence and point to the low rate of profit that they make on each sale. They do not mention, however, that a small profit for each sale made over a massive amount of sales adds up to big money. They also point to major supermarket chains, such as A&P, that are having financial trouble. But these problems are due to the inefficiency of giant corporations. In the words of the same congressional report, "...A&P stands as a monument of a conglomerate firm [i.e. a corporation that is involved in many different areas of business] with many inefficient operations that have survived because of its conglomerate power."[5]

But discovering who the culprits are is not enough for a good detective. You must also learn how they commit their crimes. The retail food industry uses many techniques that ensure that you do not have complete control over your purchasing decisions. Advertised specials are often used to bring in shoppers who then buy other products that are not on sale, and often the special is not available when the shopper arrives at the store. This practice is illegal, yet the FTC has had to order Food Fair, Shop Rite, Fisher Foods, Kroger and Safeway, among others, to make advertised specials available. If you go to the supermarket to take advantage of a special, demand it, or at least be sure that you are given a rain check.

Among other illegal practices, food stores have been caught short-weighting, adulterating products with excess water or fat and upgrading meats. (Robbins lists a number of unfair meat-retailing practices that have been found at Safeway, in his book *The Great American Food Scandal.*) One government study found that 7 percent of the shopping cart items in San Francisco and Washington D.C. were mispriced at the checkout counter; three-quarters of these were overpriced.[6] So, if you have the energy, you should check the prices that are rung up on the cash register.

But more important than these and other illegal practices are the legal gimmicks stores use to rob shoppers of making informed choices. The very organization of supermarkets is used to control the shopper's hand. Studies done by market research firms for the grocery industry (particularly the "Colonial Study" funded by *Progressive Grocer,* an industry journal) and by home economists provide insight into this process.[7] The average supermarket stocks 10,000 items. Studies show that almost half of the food purchases are unplanned and that the average shopper passes 317 items each minute, spotting a product and deciding to buy it in less than a second. As a result, store managers have lots of opportunity to manipulate your purchasing decisions.

They spread staples throughout the store, so that on the way to the salt and ketchup, for example, you have to pass the rows of shelves displaying hundreds of other products. Sales of products increase when the products are moved from floor to waist level, and increase even more when they are moved from waist to eye level, so store managers place high-profit items that lend themselves to impulse buying, like candy packaged in snack portions, at your eye level. Items appealing to children are placed, of course, on lower shelves. Thus, a good detective will look down for bargains but you have to be an acrobat to be able to spot the low-profit items placed at the level of your ankles while simultaneously distracting your child from the brightly-packaged, highly sugared, well-advertised junk food placed at his or her eye level.

If the manager wants to push an item he can place it in an end-aisle display where many shoppers will be sure to see it, and some will believe it is on sale. Sales of products moved to end-aisle displays increased over six-fold in one study. As end-aisle items are often not on sale it is always wise to check to see if a similar product at a lower price can be found on the shelves of the regular aisles.

The manager can also place candy, gum, and magazines by the checkout counter where tired, bored shoppers, their resistance broken down by an hour of shopping, will succumb to the temptation to toss those high-impulse items into their carts while waiting in line.

Product spotters (signs highlighting selected products) have been found to more than double sales by attracting shoppers' attention and sometimes falsely suggesting a bargain. Multiple pricing (three for 99¢ instead of 33¢ each) also increases sales. There is even a science of changing prices. *Progressive Grocer* advised managers to leave old price stickers showing when lowering prices. When raising prices, managers were advised to obliterate the former price and to make the change when the store is closed.[8]

The best time to avoid being manipulated by tricks like these is before you go to the store, by making a list of items you need, and by sticking to it when shopping. Unfortunately, the food industry can manipulate you even when you plan your purchases. For example, the packages that encase your food can complicate your choices between different brands of the same products.

Packaging

Packaging serves many purposes. Sometimes it protects the food. But if protection were its only purpose, much of the 600 pounds of packaging bought by the average American (up from 400 pounds in the late 1950s) would be superfluous.[9] When you cannot explain why something happens, it often pays to ask "What is in it for industry?" In the case of packaging there is more than one answer.

Some packaging, like the cardboard and cellophane used on fresh produce, encourages you to buy eight apples when you only wanted five and permits the use of brand names. As a result, although the average American consumed less fresh produce in 1970 than in 1950, the packaging encasing this produce increased by almost half in that period.[10] Isn't it comforting to know that even though you are purchasing less fresh fruit than you used to, the supermarkets are still willing to increase the amount of cardboard and cellophane that they sell you with the fruit?

Packages allow the food industry to conceal the addition of low-quality products, ingredients, and adulterants. Don't you wish that you could reject the bad strawberries hidden in the bottom of the basket? The industry also sometimes misleads you by reducing the content of a package over time without reducing the package size. In one study, cited by Ralph Nader and Beverly Moore, FDA inspectors found many packages to have high proportions of unfilled space.[11] Packages of cake and candy mixes had over one-sixth empty space. Packages of some cookies, spaghetti, and mint candies were over one-fourth empty and packages of dried desserts were almost half empty.

The lack of standard package sizes also makes it difficult for consumers to make informed choices about which product to buy. For example, only the sharpest detectives (or those with calculators) can determine the lowest price per ounce of sardines which come in three and a quarter ounce, three and three-quarter ounce, and four and three-eighths ounce cans; or of black pepper sold in one ounce, one and three-eighths ounce, one and three-quarters ounce, and two ounce containers; or coffee which comes in two, four, eight, ten, twelve, thirteen, sixteen, or thirty-two ounce jars, with the largest not necessarily being the lowest in unit price.

The packaging problem is not simply one of industry deception and consumer confusion. Eight cents out of every dollar you spend on food goes for packaging (more for some products).[12] The effects of packaging are also environmental, since packaging materials account for over one third of municipal solid waste. Each year, McDonalds alone destroys hundreds of square miles of forest for its paper packaging.[13] Energy is used to produce the packaging material and some of it, plastic for example, is made from petroleum, so, according to one estimate, if the United States could return to its 1958 level of packaging it would reduce its total energy consumption by almost one-tenth.[14]

Price Confusion

One effect of the store managers' tricks and the multiplicity of packages is general confusion about food prices. Of sixty staple items presented in the Colonial Study, the price on only one, a six-pack of Coke, was remembered by most of the people tested.[15] Supermarket confusion is best exemplified in three different studies, one performed by the California Consumer Council, one by a psychologist, and one by Consumers Union, in which shoppers were given a list of specific products to buy and told to choose solely on the basis of the most product for the lowest price. In each study, although participants had only one concern—price—and knew that their performance would be evaluated, about half of the purchases were not the best buy.[16] Imagine how many pricing errors the average shopper, who is not participating in a study, must make.

The shopper's confusion is not due to stupidity. When offered accurate, comprehensible information, consumers make use of it, as a clever piece of Canadian research shows.[17] The researchers collected prices of staple food items in twenty-six Ottawa supermarkets. When the prices were published in local newspapers, giving shoppers an easy way to compare competing prices, the difference between the prices in the most expensive and the least expensive store dropped by half. Average prices for the area declined about 7 percent. When the prices stopped being published, average prices went up again. The program cost $875 a week and saved shoppers $40,000. A follow-up study over a longer period produced similar, though less dramatic, results. Imagine how much easier shopping would be if a program like this one were instituted in every town and you could really let your fingers do the walking.

Labels

But the detective job would not be finished even if you could discover how much you are paying for food, for it would then be time to investigate the labels to discover what you are getting for your money. Food labels contain attractive pictures of colorful, tasty-looking dishes teeming with the most expensive ingredients in the recipe, that bear little relation to the actual package contents. They offer you the opportunity to send away for piggy banks, or toy submarines that will submerge in your child's bath. They provide great literature about cookie monsters or about the invention of corn. They tell you of the other products made by the company that put out the label and supply you with recipes that combine two or three of these products to create exotic, tasty dishes of the marshmallow, baked beans, American cheese surprise variety.

More important is what labels do not tell you. Food labels contain no information about the empty space in the package or the amount of water in the can or the exact proportion of each ingredient in the product. How much grape is in Welch's grape jelly? How much peanut is in Jif peanut butter? How much beef is in Libby's Beef Stew? The labels don't tell you.

Sometimes the USDA grade of a product is listed but the grading system is so needlessly complex that you cannot easily use the information. For example, if you were to buy grade A Swiss cheese you would be getting the top quality Swiss. But if you were to buy grade A cheddar cheese you would be getting the second-best cheddar—USDA top-grade cheddar is labelled AA. If consumers were able to convince the USDA to institute a sane grading system many food manufacturers would be displeased, for the system would allow you to select food based on quality rather than on brand name.

The labeling laws allow the manufacturers to leave hundreds of ingredients off the labels. If in the official food standards of the FDA an ingredient is listed as "optional," it must be mentioned on the label. But if the ingredient is listed as "permissible" for a particular kind of food, it need not be mentioned. As a result, there is no way, short of doing a chemical analysis, for anyone but the manufacturer to know exactly what indgredients are included in most foods. Sometimes the laws mandate that an ingredient be listed on the labels of some foods but not others. Emulsifying agents, for example, must be listed on pasteurized, processed food but not on pasteurized, processed cheese. In addition, some ingredients are included on labels only in vague, general categories like "batter and breading ingredients" mentioned on breaded shrimp labels.

Labels can mislead in other ways, too. One victory for consumers was the passage of legislation forcing food processors to list the ingredients in order of proportion in the recipe. But what is a shopper to make of a list of ingredients like that on Lipton Tomato Cup of Soup, which contains both "corn syrup" (a sweetener) and "sugar," or on Skippy peanut butter, which contains both "dextrose" (a type of sugar) and "sugar," or on Post Sugar Crisps, which contains "sugar," "corn syrup," "honey," and "caramel coloring," or on Campbell's Old Fashioned Beans, which contains "invert sugar," "molasses," "brown sugar," "corn syrup," "sugar," and "apple concentrate." What would the labels of these (and many other) products look like if all of the sweeteners were combined, allowing you to discover if you are buying mostly sugar?

The food industry fights against labeling legislation. Industry spokespersons testifying before Congressional committees have proposed voluntary programs, tried to eliminate the labeling of vitamin and mineral content and fought the inclusion on the label of the exact proportion of each ingredient in the product. They do this, sometimes, in the name of helping others. For example, a representative of the National Food Processors Association recommended to Congress the use of labels for promotional purposes rather than for nutrition information, ostensibly because smaller canners cannot afford large advertising budgets.[18] How considerate of the giant processors to worry so much about their small competitors. He also wanted to avoid or eliminate requirements for much nutrition information because the current labels carry too much information for consumers to absorb. We can all sleep a little bit better at night knowing that the industry that gives us sixteen package sizes of breakfast cereals and fifty-six sizes of crackers and cookies[19] is concerned that we not be overloaded with information about the package contents.

In order to make these contents match as closely as possible the pretty pictures on the label, manufacturers use dyes, preservatives, thickeners, and emulsifiers. Many foods, naturally tasty and nutritious though they may be, simply do not look as pretty as their Madison Avenue versions. Other foods, their appearance ravaged by modern farming and processing practices, require sprucing up to appear appetizing. The industry solution to these problems is "better living through chemistry."

Frankfurters would be an unappetizing grey if it were not for Orange B dye. Some oranges, greenish yellow in their natural state, look orange only because growers inject Citrus Red #2 in the rinds. Colorants in butter are added in winter to mask the natural grey-white of cream from under-nourished cows so it matches the rich yellow of more nutritious cream from cows fed on nutrient-rich grass in the summer.

Most dyes used are derived from coal tar. Between 1940 and 1971, the amount of these dyes certified for use in food by the FDA increased tenfold for each person in the United States.[20] Many of these dyes have been inadequately tested for safety. As soon as a dye like Red #2 was found to possibly cause cancer and was taken off the market, it was replaced by Red #40 which has not yet been adequately tested for the same problem. Even the Violet #1 formerly used to stamp USDA grades on meat was eventually outlawed for health reasons by the FDA.[21]

Perhaps using chemicals to make food pretty is not such a good idea, but how about using them to keep food fresh? Since spoiled food benefits no one, don't preservatives serve a useful function? The answer is certainly "yes," but the more germane question is, useful to whom?

The growth of the food industry from small, local farms and factories to large, centralized farms and factories means that today, in transit from soil to mouth, food must pass through grain elevators, processing plants, wholesalers, supermarket warehouses, and market shelves, before reaching your home, not to mention all of the trains, trucks and storage in between. As a result, a great deal of time elapses between the moment when food crops are harvested and the moment you eat them.

To prevent the food from decaying even before you buy it, the food industry monkeys around with it. Tomatoes are picked unripe, then gas-ripened. Tuna is canned, often using lead solder, which has produced lead contamination in tuna up to 10,000 times the naturally occurring level.[22] Meat spoilage is reduced by introducing sodium nitrite, a potential carcinogen (i.e. cause of cancer) which is used in part because it gives meat an appetizing reddish hue. Butylated hydroxyanisole (BHA) and butylated hydroxytoluene (BHT) are used in products containing oil, even though Eastern Chemical Products, a major producer of these chemicals, has admitted that "BHA and/or BHT are not found to provide significant improvement in the...stability of vegetable oils."[23]

Of course, some chemical goodies do keep food from spoiling once you bring it home, and some seem relatively harmless in the quantities used by food processors. But, in the average household, a major shopping trip is made once a week.[24] Most foods will not go bad in that time. Those items that cannot last a week, like freshly baked bread, could be sold in small stores located near most homes, schools and workplaces, enabling people to easily pick them up almost every day. Methods of preservation that are slower but healthier than the chemical methods used by the food industry, such as pickling and drying, have been around for centuries and could be used, when necessary, today. So, were it not for the highly-centralized organization of the farms, factories and super-markets, many of you could do without most of the chemicals used to preserve food, with very little inconvenience. The preservatives put into food are there not so much to preserve the food in your home as to preserve the profits and concentration of power of the food industry.

Perhaps you believe that while extensive processing and shipping may have disadvantages, they at least allow you to have great variety in your diet. In support of this notion industry spokespeople point to the thousands of "new" food items that have appeared in the last few years. The American consumer does have access to some foodstuffs—anchovies from Peru, instant coffee, ocean fish in the Midwest and pineapples in Minnesota—that were not readily available in the past, except in some cases to wealthy customers. Included among these are some radically new products.

According to the USDA's John Connor,[25] however, almost all of the "new" products are either imitations (e.g. Schlitz Lite copied Anheuser Natural Light), line extensions (Kellogg Bran Buds added to an already extensive line of bran cereals), reformulations (Morton's New Lemon Cream Pie finally includes lemons), or repositions (baby foods sold as quick snacks for adults). In other words, they are not really new products. And there is not always an obvious need for some of the products that are really new, like Cumberland Butter Buds—synthetic butter that cannot be used for frying or spreading. Thus, much of the apparent variety in supermarkets is simply a profusion of subtly varying clones in markedly different packages, or "new" products that you did not need in the first place.

The proliferation of products not only gives a false impression of variety, it is also wasteful. The ads and promotions necessary for introducing a new product are expensive, and their effects are often cancelled by competitors who boost their own ad spending. Introducing new products is risky, representing gambles of million dollar magnitude. And new products tend to be more expensive. Light beer, for example, is cheaper to produce than regular beer but sells for higher prices.

Product proliferation allows companies to change products slightly rather than lowering prices or improving quality. It also allows large companies able to offer full product lines to crowd the products of smaller producers off the supermarket shelves, promoting concentration within the food manufacturing industry. The resultant profits are used for advertising and for further product proliferation.

Most of the food marketing problems that have been discussed so far are particularly bad for poor people. In the United States, the poor are in a double bind—not only do they have less money to buy the food they need, they also have to pay higher prices for food (and many other goods). Many government studies find that because low-income neighborhoods have fewer supermarkets than other neighborhoods, poor people must shop at small independent stores. In today's world of giant corporations, these small stores cannot get the same deals from suppliers as do large supermarket chains, so they have to charge more than do the supermarkets. The lack of supermarkets means that there is also less competition in low-income areas so stores in these areas can get away with more than can stores in wealthier neighborhoods. Advertised specials were found to be twice as likely to be unavailable in low-income areas of Washington, D.C. as in high-income areas.[26] Poor people also get lower-quality food. The USDA found that three times as many samples of ground beef bought in stores in low-income areas had excess fat compared to samples bought in high-income areas.[27]

The FTC summarized these findings:

> Many foodstores serving low-income, inner-city areas are small, less efficient and have higher prices. Consumers in these areas are frequently sold lower quality merchandise and are provided fewer services than in other areas. Moreover, the retail facilities of low-income areas are often old and in a shabby state of upkeep.[28]

The inequity is not limited to major cities. A survey of a Tennessee community revealed that, whereas most people shop at supermarkets, most food stamp recipients cannot because they live farther from supermarkets and have less access to transportation.[29]

Although some people accuse the poor of spending public assistance dollars on luxury items, there is evidence that poor Americans economize wisely to adapt to their adverse conditions. A USDA study found that low-income households stretch their food dollars by buying less-costly meats and fewer snacks than higher-income families. Another USDA study found that low-income households get more nutrition for each food dollar than do their wealthier counterparts.

For a variety of reasons stores in nonpoverty areas show twice as much profit per sales dollar as poverty-area stores.[30] Therefore, given a system of food for profit, it makes sense for supermarket chains to avoid low-income areas. But how sensible is a food system if it ends up charging the most for food to the people who can least afford it? And how sensible is the food marketing system we now have that overcharges consumers, manipulates shoppers by intentionally confusing them about what they are paying and what they are getting, and adds chemicals to foods to make them easier to market?

The answer would seem to be obvious but what can you do about it? In addition to studying the traps set by the food industry in an attempt to avoid them, you can learn about the several alternatives that have cropped up to skirt the problems of profit-centered supermarkets, including food co-ops, direct marketing, and political action by consumers.

Food co-ops are responsive to consumers because they are consumer owned. Profits are of secondary importance to service, and any profits made are returned to co-op members in dividends. Two large, successful co-ops illustrate the benefits of co-oping: The Consumers Cooperative of Berkeley Inc. in California, and Greenbelt Consumer Services Inc. in Greenbelt, Maryland. The Berkeley Co-op has a chain of twelve stores. The Greenbelt Co-ops have six supermarkets, two produce stores, and a network of other businesses unrelated to food.

Both co-ops emphasize marketing for service, not for profit. They do not rely on end-aisle displays of junk food or impulse items. They employ price policies that guarantee lower unit prices for large packages than for small packages. They sell in bulk items like whole grains, beans, and fresh produce. They emphasize direct marketing, the sale of unpacked goods to minimize labor charges and maximize freshness. Finally, both co-ops emphasize consumer education.

The Berkeley Co-op stresses consumer education through staff home economists who counsel on nutrition by putting informative signs in the stores and by publishing a weekly newsletter. In cooperation with these specialists, merchandisers have stopped advertising highly-sugared cereals, sell fewer of them, and display only the bottoms of the cereal packages to minimize their visual impact. Store ads emphasize nutritious sale items presented with information about nutrients, cooking instructions, and storage. The co-op sells items not readily available from other local stores, such as nitrite-free hot dogs. The co-op also has a consumer protection committee to lobby on food issues and work with local action groups.

The Greenbelt Co-op also emphasizes conscientious marketing policies, like unit pricing, open dating, and nutritional labeling. Less oriented toward health food than Berkeley, it supplies a more extensive range of goods and services to its members, including service stations with discount gas, a credit union, and group legal services.

Many consumers take advantage of direct marketing, buying food from farmers at farmers' markets, green markets, and direct marketing farms. Buying directly from farmers ensures that the money in your food budget goes to feed you, not the middlemen and is a good way of reducing food spoilage without using preservatives. More than half of the farms in New Jersey, for example, sold directly to consumers in 1978.[31] In Michigan that year, apples alone accounted for more than ten million dollars in direct marketing sales. In addition to fruits and vegetables, farmers sell flowers and plants, meat and poultry, honey, dairy products, nuts, and seasonal products like Christmas trees.

Many people throughout the country have formed buying clubs that purchase food in bulk from farmers or wholesalers and distribute it to club members. Each member usually commits a few hours each month to shopping for, transporting or distributing the food. In return they obtain fresh food at bargain prices.

People dissatisfied with our current food marketing system have also set up farmers' markets in their communities, organized to change the foods available from vending machines at their schools or workplaces and worked on returnable container campaigns. In 1981 the New York Public Interest Research Group spearheaded a fight that resulted in a law mandating returnable beverage containers in Suffolk County, New York. In 1974 one consumers group in Buffalo was able to successfully fight the test marketing of a sugary, fat-laden new General Mills cereal in Buffalo supermarkets.

The alternative marketing systems demonstrate that the root of the marketing problems detailed in this chapter is the antagonistic relationship set up between buyer and seller in a distribution system based on profits for industry. Gimmicks, confusing packaging and labeling, high prices for poor people, along with other gyps and swindles occur when sellers must liberate the most money possible from the customer at the least expense to themselves. The marketplace in a "free enterprise" system is supposed to be the place where buyers and sellers meet and as everyone pursues their own self-interest—buyers trying to get the most for the least and sellers trying to give the least for the most—everyone benefits. But this description is a lie. It does not apply to the modern food market (nor, for that matter, to the rest of the American economy). The high concentration of all parts of the system means that a few powerful sellers have an unfair advantage when bargaining with many customers. The complex processing and tricky merchandising techniques used by the food industry make it almost impossible for consumers to be informed as to which products are best, again giving an unfair advantage to the corporations. Finally, advertising puts even more power in the hands of the food industry, as you will see in Chapter 6.

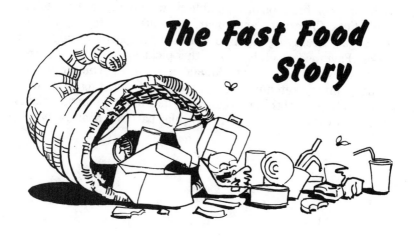

The Fast Food Story

Franchised fast food is the next step after convenience food. The food is not only prepared for you, it is also heated and served, using the assembly line production methods preferred by industry.

Most of the largest restaurant chains are fast food corporations. Sales of fast food equal about $20 billion.[1] In 1978 McDonalds alone had sales of over $4 billion.[2] McDonalds buys one percent of the beef wholesaled in the United States and is the nation's largest purchaser of fish, having made its owner, Ray Kroc, one of the richest people in the country.[3] Other fast food chains were not quite so powerful and were bought out by large food conglomerates. Burger King was acquired by Pillsbury, Burger Chef by General Foods, Jack in the Box by Ralston-Purina, Kentucky Fried Chicken by Heublein, Pizza Hut by Pepsico, Arby's by RC Cola, and A&W by United Brands. The problems with fast foods are similar to those with convenience foods. They are expensive. Five quarter pounders purchased in 1981 at a McDonalds in New York State averaged less than a fifth of a pound, without the bun or any trimmings, and cost $1.35. That is $7.50 per pound of meat. Even if we take into account some shrinkage during cooking and the cost of the other ingredients, the price of fast food beef greatly exceeds the $1.79 a pound at the supermarket near the McDonalds. The USDA reported that a meal consisting of a special hamburger, french fries, and a soft drink cost almost twice as much in a fast food restaurant as it would at home.[4]

Fast food meals are not very nutritious. According to nutritionist Jean Mayer they are low in vitamins B and C and high in saturated fat.[5] The shakes are not made with whole milk but rather with some combination of vegetable oil, casein, nonfat milk solids, emulsifiers, flavorings, and sugar. They are high in fat, calories, and sugar, averaging eight to fourteen teaspoons of sugar per shake.[6] Fast food vegetables are either pickles, tomatoes, or frozen french fries (unless you are Ronald Reagan, in which case you would count the ketchup as a vegetable). Many fast foods are high in salt. There is nothing wrong with fast foods as an occasional snack, but they are not good as a regular part of a healthy diet.

Food Preparation
and the Family

A can of soup that can be warmed up fast after walking home from school on a freezing cold day. An extra jar of spaghetti sauce when friends drop by unexpectedly. A bag of nuts discovered in the cupboard just as the late movie starts. That old, dear, reliable friend, the tuna fish sandwich. These things may not be the bedrock upon which modern civilization is built, but they do make life a bit more pleasant. Cooking for a few hours can be fun on occasion, but not always, and it is not always feasible. Everyone would agree that it is possible for a human being to be simultaneously hungry and either tired, lazy, busy, or in a hurry, so it is no big deal if here and there we open a can or box when we want a quick and easy meal.

But the food industry takes advantage of our desire for convenience to promote the overuse of processed foods. "Do you want to keep homemakers chained to their stoves?" its spokespeople ask advocates of fresh food. "Maybe you have a fetish for the nineteenth century or can't handle our modern, fast-paced lifestyle" they insinuate. These accusations serve to justify the need for profitable prepared foods.

But what about convenience? Don't we need processed foods to make our lives easier? What is wrong with having the food industry take some of the burden off busy people? What alternatives are there to convenience foods?

Obviously some convenience products are really convenient and nobody would want to do away with all of them. This statement is not as silly as it sounds because some convenience foods are not really much more convenient than the foods they replace. Instant omelettes, for example, are very easy to use. You open the container, pour the contents into a pan, and cook up an omelette. Compare this no-bother method to the troublesome ordinary method of making an omelette in which you crack open a couple of eggs, beat them slightly after adding a little milk, pour them into a pan and perhaps throw in some mushrooms or cheese. Another real labor savor is boil-in-bag spaghetti which allows you to simply drop a pouch into boiling water instead of actually having to touch the spaghetti.

These are extreme examples, but many common prepared foods save much less time than the food industry would have you believe. Is opening a box of Green Giant broccoli in butter sauce, removing the pouch, dropping the pouch into boiling water, taking it out of the water, splitting it open, and emptying the contents onto a plate, much faster or easier than cutting up a stalk of broccoli, tossing it into a steamer that is resting in a pot of boiling water, removing the pieces, and putting on some butter and pepper? And is it really that difficult to make an herb dressing by combining three-quarters cup of oil, three tablespoons of vinegar, one-quarter teaspoon of dry mustard, one-half teaspoon of basil, two teaspoons of chives, and a teaspoon each of salt, tarragon, and chervil, rather than buying a bottled salad dressing? Is heating a TV dinner so much faster and easier than broiling or baking fresh meat, poultry, or fish, and boiling a potato? Some convenience foods save you a lot of trouble, but by no means all.

Being processed, convenience foods are usually expensive. Pancake mixes are a good example. For one cent a pancake, (1982 New York price) you can buy Pillsbury "Extra Light" Hungry Jack Pancake Mix to which you add eggs, milk, and shortening in order to make pancake batter. For two cents a pancake, Pillsbury will add the ingredients for you, you need only add water. For six cents a pancake, Aunt Jemima will see to it that you just have to pour the batter into a pan. If that is too much work, for ten cents a pancake, you can pop precooked Downy Flake pancakes into the toaster. And if you're really looking for convenience, for twenty-six cents a pancake, you can heat in your oven Swanson pancakes onto which the syrup has already been poured.

When the convenience foods appear to cost as little per serving as homemade meals, it is usually because they contain much less of the higher-priced, more nutritious ingredients than do home cooked foods. When dieticians compared the ingredients in prepared foods with those in typical home cooked meals, as represented by USDA homemade recipes, they found that a serving of canned chicken chow mein contains one-tenth an ounce of chicken, and a serving of frozen chicken chow mein contains one-half an ounce, while the USDA homemade recipe contains two and one-third ounces.[1] Canned beef stew contains beef, carrots, and potatoes. The homemade recipe included these ingredients as well as peas and onions. The cheese in canned spaghetti is romano and cheddar, which are cheaper than the parmesan cheese in the homemade recipe.

Thus, convenience foods cost more, are less healthy, or are more fattening (see Chapter 9) than fresh foods. And while a selective use of convenience foods can make life easier, with a few simple recipes, a little bit of confidence, and a lot of resistance to advertisements, most of us could cut down drastically on our use of these items without spending much extra time cooking.

But as long as we can afford very little time for food preparation, we will be forced to rely on too many convenience foods. In order to understand how this state of affairs came to be, why it is not inevitable, and why the overuse of convenience foods is not our fault, we have to understand a bit about the history of the American family.

The Family

Families have always been linked to the economic and social structures of society. The family fulfills some economic functions, and economic changes in a society lead to changes in the role played by the family and to changes in family structure. For example, when the economy was based primarily on agriculture, the family was the unit responsible for most economic tasks, including the growth and preparation of food and the production of other necessities, like shelter and clothing.

On a farm, many hands are needed and there are tasks that can be done by people ranging in age from very young to very old. And in the preindustrial period, there was less geographic mobility than there is today. As a result, the members of many farm families— parents, children, grandparents, aunts, uncles, cousins—lived in close proximity, and most of them worked to produce the basic necessities of life. Men and women, young and old, worked together to survive. So, compared to modern families, the members of many preindustrial families lived closer to one another, shared more tasks, and were more involved in the production of the goods necessary for subsistence. Even in the early days of industrialism, much of the production of goods for sale that occurred both in the home and in the early shops that were the precursors of factories was done by families working together, usually under the supervision of the father.

The development of a private profit industrial economic system, however, removed production from the control of families and centralized it in large corporate units. Thus, the corporation, centered in the factory, not the family, centered in the home, became the basic economic unit. The economic role played by the family and its members changed.

At first, although the skilled crafts were controlled by men, many of the industrial wage workers were women and children working in the textile industry.[2] Over time, however, men came to make up the bulk of the industrial workers, partly because of laws that limited the hours worked by women and children,[3] and partly because men monopolized the jobs in heavy industry—iron, steel, machinery—which, due to the growth of the railroads, became the most numerous jobs.

Thus, by late nineteenth century, the situation had become one in which most men went to work outside the home, while most (but by no means all) women stayed at home rearing children, taking care of the home and of daily health care, and preparing food. This housework included important tasks that were necessary for the maintenance of life and integral to the workings of the economy. But, in a private profit system everything is valued based on the profit it produces, and although housework was necessary, it was not profitable, so it became devalued. Women were not producing profit, so they were not paid wages, so they came to be thought of as not really working and as contributing less to society. Recent economic changes have allowed for, and even promoted the increased employment of women outside of the home. Industry developed a need for cheaper labor, particularly labor that would work part-time and that could be convinced to stop working and return to the home in times of high unemployment. Mechanization took place. The number of clerical jobs increased as shipping, advertising, and marketing became more important. More effective contraception was developed as children went from being sources of help on the farms and in the shops to being economic burdens, so women had to spend less time having and caring for children. Inflation made it more difficult for many families to get by on one salary. And the need for growth led the corporations, including the food industry, to search for new areas of investment.

Businesses had already taken over most of the production work previously done in and around the home, so, to continue growing, they had to take over and make profitable the previously free services provided by women as housework. "Women's work," including teaching, counselling, health care, and food preparation, have increasingly become jobs performed for wages. The home has become mainly a place to bring up children and to "get away from it all." Over hundreds of years, a division has developed (uncommon in agricultural societies) between work and family life, and the economic role of the family has changed from the production of basic necessities to the production of new workers and the consumption of marketed goods. So, American families have changed from agricultural families working together to grow and prepare food and other necessities, to families in which dad goes out to work and comes back home to relax and eat dinner with the wife and kids, to families whose members all go their separate ways and probably do not even eat together most days, to single, separated, widowed, or divorced people who now constitute about a quarter of all households. Ironically, those people who are most upset by these changes tend to be the ones who are the staunchest defenders of the economic system that has produced the changes.

The advantages of some of the changes are obvious. Women working for wages have more control over some aspects of their lives than they used to, and they may be less financially dependent on men than they were. The idea that women are human beings worthy of treatment equal to that given men is, in part, based on women's participation in the profit economy. But the disadvantages are also striking. The jobs that most women can get are, on the average, lower paying and lower in prestige than are men's jobs. Women are also placed in a double bind; they must work, but they are usually still responsible for at least overseeing their old tasks of homemaking, childrearing, and food preparation. In some ways they are worse off than they used to be, and in the average household there is less time available for the preparation of food.

Food Preparation

The organization and timing of people's jobs define the organization and timing of their lives, and the organization of work nowadays is not designed to promote adequate food preparation. By the time most people return from nine to five jobs, they have neither much time nor much energy for shopping and cooking. If our society were designed to promote health and happiness, the influx of women into the workplace might have produced beneficial changes in the lives of everyone. The system wherein men worked forty hours a week to earn incomes while women worked long hours bringing up children, cleaning house, and preparing meals, might have been replaced by a system wherein both adults worked outside of the home for, say, twenty-five hours, and both shared the tasks of homemaking (along with their children). This would reduce the number of hours any one person would have to work at any one job, either outside or inside the home. It would also increase the time spent by fathers with their children, and increase the total number of hours of wage labor by family members—from forty hours for one person to fifty hours for two—thus increasing (if wages were fair) the total family income. Finally, it would allow more time for preparing meals, reducing even more the need for convenience foods, and thus reducing expenses.

But, rather than changing the organization and timing of work and redistributing homemaking tasks among all family members, many of the tasks have been put into the hands of industry, continuing the trend of turning private social tasks into profitable business transactions. After some industries had hired women at low wages to do what they had been previously doing in the home, thus reducing the time that could be used by adult family members for their own and their families' needs, the food industry was able to sell back the results of some of this labor for a profit. The convenience food industry blossomed as part of the new consumer society. All that was needed to complete the picture was a means of training people to become modern consumers. And so we turn to advertising.

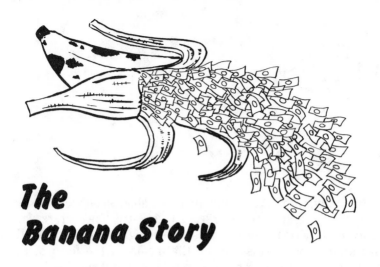

The Banana Story

In the 1960s the United Fruit Company decided to take advantage of consumer willingness to pay more for advertised brand-name items. Although United Fruit's bananas were no different from other bananas, they adorned their fruit with cute labels and dubbed it "Chiquita."

To give consumers the idea that this fruit was superior, an advertising campaign was launched stressing qualities that customers would find difficult to verify at the market. The first claim was that Chiquitas kept longer than other bananas, but people soon began to notice that wasn't true. Then the claim was made that Chiquitas bruised less than other bananas, but complaints about bruising began to roll in. The campaign finally began to succeed when it turned to assertions that Chiquitas were simply of higher quality than other bananas.

A consumer survey found that 49 percent of the women interviewed looked for Chiquitas when shopping, and 25 percent were willing to go to another store to find Chiquitas if the first store they searched didn't carry the brand.

United Fruit had created a preference and was able to charge ninety-seven cents more per box of Chiquitas than for the company's other unbranded bananas.

Based on an account from William Robbins' *The American Food Scandal,* New York: William Morrow & Co., Inc., 1974

Advertising

Traditionally, information and attitudes about food were passed down from generation to generation. Currently, however, responsibility for nutrition information is increasingly assumed by public institutions—by schools and by the media in the form of advertising. The latter is perhaps the most important single source of consumer opinion about food.

Natural limitations in human need and capacity for food are double-edged: they are a blessing for the average person and a curse for food industrialists, whose wealth and power depend on their ability to sell as much as possible.

Until the late nineteenth century, the American economy focused mainly on production. The problem was to grow or produce enough goods to meet the needs of the population. But, by the late 1800s conditions had changed to a situation in which the basic needs of most Americans could be relatively easily met by the available farms and factories.

The early American settlers and the immigrants who later streamed into the country had been brought up to be thrifty and hard-working. These attitudes made people productive but not very interested in purchasing manufactured goods. Business interests came to realize that their sales, and hence their profits, would level off unless they could change these attitudes.

The food industry's "problem" of limited demand for its products was manageable when there were many new mouths to feed, during years of booming population growth. But once population growth slowed, the problem of limited demand might have become catastrophic if it weren't for a revolutionary idea: advertising. In the words of one proponent, advertising is "the only institution we have for instilling new needs" and allows the citizen to "be educated to perform his [sic] role as a consumer, especially as a consumer of goods for which he feels no impulse or need."[1]

What an innovative idea! If old needs are limited, create new ones. Use the extensive resources of industry to support a massive

74

propaganda effort. Convince people that consumption is the answer to many of their problems and show them all of the opportunities to consume that they may be missing. When they have consumed all of the old products, new products and new needs can be created.

Sound difficult? It's not really. For example, up until the mid-1970s, many people were shirking their roles as consumers by drinking water, free and cold, from the tap. Heavy advertising campaigns, however, built bottled mineral water into an $111 million industry by 1979, with sales having increased 640 percent in just the three years since 1976.[2]

Instances like this one raise doubts that poor dietary and purchasing habits come from consumer ignorance alone, although spokespeople for the food industry would like to create that impression. The picture they paint goes something like this: "We food industry folks just give the public what it wants; we cater to public need." The consumer becomes an updated Adam whose Original Sin is choosing apple pie over apples, and whose descendants are doomed to congenital inability to learn about or practice good eating habits.

But the very nature of advertising belies this fable. According to a definition which won a contest run by the major trade newspaper *Advertising Age*, advertising is "the dissemination of information concerning an idea, service, or product to compel action in accordance with the intent of the advertiser."[3] "The intent of the advertiser" is not primarily to educate but to increase profits and expand the market. And profit, as we've already seen, means skimping on food quality while maximizing prices.

Corporations Involved in the Food Industry That Spent Over $200 million on Advertising in 1980[4]		
Corporation	Total ad budget ($ millions)	Major foods advertised
Proctor & Gamble	649.6	Folgers coffee, Pringles potato chips
General Foods	410.0	Jell-O, Maxwell House, Post cereals
Phillip Morris	364.6	Miller beer, 7-Up
R.J. Reynolds	298.5	Del Monte, Chun King Hawaiian Punch
Warner Lambert	235.2	Entenmanns, Trident gum
Gulf & Western	233.8	Schraffts
PepsiCo	233.4	Pepsi, Frito-Lay, Pizza Hut
McDonalds	207.0	Burgers, fries, etc.
Ralston Purina	206.8	Jack in the Box, Chicken of the Sea, Cookie Crisp

Scene:

You are sitting at home watching television when a commercial comes on. On the screen you see a few cans. Some are closed, exhibiting their labels, and others are open, exhibiting their contents. Next to the cans are a few prepared dishes. The announcer begins to speak:

Hello. I'd like to tell you about Blippo's canned shark. Many people find it quite tasty, particularly when it is spread on bread or crackers, or mixed with fresh vegetables and gravy, or in a salad with oil and vinegar. It contains vitamins blah, blah, and blah, and minerals blah and blah, but it is lacking in vitamins blah and blah, so it should probably be eaten in combination with blah. It contains moderately high quantities of fatty blah so it's best to avoid eating it in combination with blah. Of course, fresh fish is healthier for you, but in circumstances when fresh fish is unavailable, Blippo's canned shark is a suitable substitute if not over-used.

It may be helpful to know that the cheaper type of Blippo's canned shark is less attractive, but equally as healthy as the more expensive type. Blippo's canned shark should range in price from blah to blah, and it is available at blah. Caution: persons with heart trouble should avoid large quantities of canned shark. Others, however, should enjoy it.

Sounds ridiculous, doesn't it? Why? Perhaps because we have all internalized the idea that food advertising, like much else in our society, must be based on profit and therefore could never honestly present information like this commercial. Thus, although advertising is justified as a way to inform consumers, a truly informative ad doesn't have a chance of appearing.

In 1978, Proctor and Gamble spent $31,351,800 to advertise Folger's coffee.[5] What do you know about Folger's coffee other than that it is "mountain grown" and "It tastes as rich as it looks?" A study of children's advertising found that in addition to taste, the attributes of the products that were most frequently mentioned were size, shape, and texture; among the least frequently mentioned attributes was nutritional value.[6] Of course, advertisements do sometimes teach us valuable lessons on nutrition. After all, where else would we learn that a six-letter word for a source of vitamin C is "R-E-X-A-L-L?"

If we don't get education or accurate information in advertisements, what do we get in their place? In the words of one advertising text: "The information given in advertisements is generally only incidental to their main purpose, which is persuasion."[7]

Advertising Tricks

How do advertisers attempt to persuade us? One way is through outright deception. They substitute shaving cream for whipped cream in ads to make the topping look thicker, or put molasses in coffee to give it the appearance of more body. A brief list of some of the cases dealt with by the Federal Trade Commission in recent years includes: the charge against Campbell's Soup of putting glass marbles in the bottom of the bowls in its ads to force all of the chunky stuff to the surface; the charge against the makers of Profile bread for calling Profile a diet bread when it's only sliced thinner than other breads; the order to ITT's Continental Bakers to state in its ads that the fiber in Fresh Horizon Bread comes from wood pulp; the order to a dairy industry front called the National Commission on Egg Nutrition to cease claiming that no scientific evidence exists linking cholesterol to heart disease; the order to another industry front, the Vitamin Education Institute, to cease making unsubstantiated weight-loss claims for its vitamins; and the order to Richard's Foods to cease claiming directly or by implication that Fearn Natural Soya Powder is an adequate substitute for cows' milk for infants less than one year old.[8]

These are just some of the deceptions uncovered by the FTC. But deception is just the tip of the iceberg. Sometimes ads can mislead by leaving out information rather than by fabricating directly. One ad states that in a survey, kids with a preference picked Peter Pan peanut butter over Jif or Skippy. The ad doesn't say how many kids had a preference. So, as a hypothetical example, out of 100 kids surveyed, fifty-five may have had no preference, eighteen may have preferred Peter Pan, sixteen may have preferred Jif, and eleven may have preferred Skippy. Big deal! The point is that with only the information available from the ad there is no way of knowing whether to drop everything and run to the store for some Peter Pan.

Perhaps more harmful are the bizarre assumptions and crazy attitudes about food and eating purveyed by advertisements that the average person may begin to believe after being bombarded by ads day and night, on radio and tv, in newspapers and magazines, and on highways, buses, and trains. One commercial shows the members of a family hurriedly leaving home in the morning without eating. The mother, who doesn't seem to be going anywhere, commiserates with the women in the tv audience on the difficulties of getting families to eat breakfast. Fortunately, she finds a solution. She leaves plates of Hostess crumb cakes and donuts in the kitchen so that her husband and kids can grab them on the way out. What a simple solution to a common problem! Of course, after years of exposure to similar commercials, we never question the advisability of starting the day with a diet of sugar. The food industry has so befuddled our minds as to be able to use a sincere concern for good eating to persuade people to buy junk foods.

Along similar lines is the Cookie Crisp commercial aimed at children that advises them to "make a cookie jar" out of their cereal bowl by eating Cookie Crisp which "looks like chocolate chip cookies, you see, but it's really a cereal that's good for you and me. Tastes like chocolate chip cookies too." The first absurdity is the idea of training kids to eat cookies for breakfast. The second is assuming that eating a cereal which contains sugar as a primary ingredient, as well as salt, corn syrup, artificial flavor, cocoa, corn starch, yellow dye #5, artificial color, and BHT is any better than eating regular cookies.

Another technique used to mislead us is the use of unexplained catchwords. We've already seen how "natural" is used to describe cheddar cheese containing artificial ingredients, and how "en-riched" is used to describe bread from which vitamins are removed. There are other instances of misused or ill-defined catchwords. We're told that Top Choice is the only dog food with that impressive-sounding ingredient "high-quality protein." In failing to explain what "high-quality protein" is or what purpose it serves, the commercial is trying to manipulate us by playing upon our ignorance of nutrition and respect for scientific terminology.

The food industry also plays on the desire for convenience. Fresh or minimally processed foods that are cheaper and healthier than the highly processed version are often just about as easy to prepare; but they don't produce as much profit, so advertisers try to convince people that they are incapable of preparing their own food. Not only does advertising promote a sense of helplessness, a feeling that the fine points of food preparation are just too difficult for mere mortals; it also creates anxiety and guilt. If people can be made to feel that they are constantly being evaluated by others against strict standards and that they could never live up to these standards without help, they can be sold millions of dollars worth of products they wouldn't otherwise buy.

The problem is that the food industry creates, or at least promotes, helplessness, anxiety, and guilt in order to sell its products. Were you constantly distracted by concern about bad breath before you were told that "Certs takes your mind off your mouth for an hour"? How much guilt over enjoyment of eating were you experiencing when Weight Watchers told you, "Now you can eat without feeling like a criminal"? How worried were you about disapproval of your cooking by friends and relatives before Minute Rice and Maxwell House began to recount tales of important dinners completely ruined by imperfect rice, and ideal marriages threatened by rotten coffee, and the cute little Pillsbury doughboy advised you to "Bake a good impression?" The point is that people who have the power to decide what to put in advertisements profit by building up the insecurities of the public.

Perhaps the main reason consumers are not completely paranoid is that advertisers can also make money by focusing on the positive. In order to get people to pick up their products during that quick trip down the supermarket aisle, advertisers try to create positive associations for the products by selling the product as part of a lifestyle. In the words of the president of an ad agency with a bottled water account:

> While others are building on a theme of heritage, we're selling Saratoga as a fashion item. We believe in utilizing people, presenting young and attractive bodies against an American landscape. We're not just selling water; it's more complex than that.[9]

Another bottled water advertiser said, "We're selling New England integrity to a broad target group."

In addition to heritage, fashion, and integrity, food advertisers sell: fun ("have a Coke and a smile"); youth ("You're in the Pepsi generation;" "Pepsi, for those who think young"); friendship ("Here's to good friends"); community ("Maxwell House is bringing folks together"); not to mention love, motherhood, nostalgia, and prestige ("Your water level should rise to your social level.")

Advertisers don't limit themselves to verbal messages. They use lush natural settings to sell highly processed foods, energetic children engaged in sports to promote devitalizing candy bars, and scenes of families enjoying good ol' home cookin' to push prepackaged, ready-made products.

Ads also sell by testimonial the way evangelists purvey religion. Celebrities are often used to give a product the right cachet. A list of celebrities that have endorsed food products would be tediously long. Perhaps the most extreme misuse of the testimonial is the promotion of junk foods by athletes, naming candies after Babe Ruth and Reggie Jackson.

But the food industry doesn't have to rely on sports and entertainment celebs to sell; it has the power to create its own celebrities. Tony the Tiger and Ronald MacDonald are just two of the characters created specifically to get children to desire certain foods. And recently, corporations, attempting to avoid the sterile, uncaring image of Big Business, have begun to use their slightly homely presidents as media images. Tom Carvel and Frank Perdue have stolen the hearts of America.

The Targets

Also enlightening are the targets at whom advertising is directed. Many food advertisers would agree with the representative of one biscuit manufacturer, who said, "Sunshine's prime target is still women eighteen to forty-nine, although children also play a big part in the purchase decision."[10] The emphasis on women is shown by a study in which we found that women's magazines contained over a hundred times as many ads for food as men's magazines.[11]

The ads themselves also perpetuate sexist and racist attitudes. In a study of 133 tv commercials aimed at kids, 124 had a major spokesperson.[12] Of these, only eleven were female—two of these were off-stage voices, three were children, five were mothers (four of whom were shown in the kitchen), and one was a waitress. A woman's place appears to be in the home, or buying food, not selling it. One teenage male of Spanish origin was the only member of a minority group to be a spokesperson.

Advertising to children is very common. One study found that on children's tv shows fifteen commercials were broadcast every hour; 60 percent or more of these commercials were for food.[13] Other studies found even higher proportions of food advertising on children's television, up to 82 percent, compared to an estimate of 25 percent on adult television. Thus, of the approximately 25,000 commercials seen by the average child each year, somewhere between 15,000 and 20,000 may be for edible items.

Why is the food industry aiming its ads at kids? There seem to be two reasons. First of all, children are less able than adults to resist advertisements or to weigh the merits of purchasing the advertised items. In one study, over half of the five to seven year old children were unaware of the selling motive of commercials.[14] A quote from an advertising trade journal from 1912, when industry spokespeople were less concerned about guarding their language, will serve to make the point:

Isn't it reasonable to suppose that if these advertisers get these facts into the minds of the children while they are young and easily impressionable, it will be pretty hard for their competitors to advertise them out of their minds after they are grown up?[15]

The result, as portrayed in a recent soup commercial, is young children who cannot spell with their alphabet soup because they haven't yet learned to spell, but who do know how to sing "Give me the Campbell life." So one reason to advertise to children is to sneak the message in before rational judgement processes are developed.

The second reason is that although children have little direct purchasing power, they sometimes have considerable indirect clout. One study of shopping practices found that over one-third of mothers of five to seven year old children usually yielded to them when purchasing snack foods, and nine out of ten mothers usually yielded when purchasing breakfast cereals.[16] If you were an advertiser out for a profit, you would be silly to miss the opportunity to sell your product to such an unsuspecting, yet influential, audience.

Luckily, there are people who are doing something about advertising on children's television. Action for Children's Television (ACT) is a nonprofit consumer organization that aims to improve broadcasting practices that affect kids. The organization began when a small group of Boston homemakers met at the home of one of them to discuss the problem of manipulative advertising directed at children. They built their small group into a national organization. Among the accomplishments of ACT are the reduction of advertising on children's weekend tv by 40 percent, the elimination of vitamin ads on kids' programs, and the elimination of the use of children's show hosts as product pushers.

They Decide What You Will Buy

Although unethical, the strategy of marketing to children might be less problematic if the food pushed on women and children were nutritious. But, alas, such is not the case. In deciding which products to advertise, the main concern of the food industry is profits.

A glance at the highly advertised products on page 75, or at almost any tv show or magazine, will quickly reveal which products are high earners. How many ads exist for fresh fruit, vegetables, or fish? Now think of all the ads for "fruit flavored" candy, gum, or sugared drinks; for highly processed vegetable products like cornflakes, potato chips, or tomato ketchup; for fried, frozen, or fast-food fish.

In 1979, the Idaho Potato Commission, one of the largest advertisers of a fresh, unprocessed product, spent roughly $1.2 million on advertising.[17] In 1978, Proctor & Gamble spent ten times that amount just to advertise Pringles Potato Chips.[18] About the only advertising which even mentions fresh corn is done by Mazola "made with the goodness of maize," while in 1978, Pepsico, owners of Frito-Lay, spent over $10 million to advertise Doritos tortilla chips.[19]

A review of seven studies of advertising on childrens' television found that the proportion of food ads that were for sugared cereals ranged from 25 percent to 42 percent; for candies and sweets, from 23 percent to 46 percent; for soft drinks and fruit drinks, from 0 percent to 9 percent (the total of all sugared foods ranged from 59 percent to 76 percent); for fast-food restaurants, from 9 percent to 23 percent; while the proportion of food ads that were for fruits and juices ranged from 0 percent to 2 percent; for milk and dairy products, from 1 percent to 2 percent; and for vegetables there were no commercials found in any of the studies.[20] In one of the studies, a detailed analysis of the food contents found that 97.9 percent of the advertised foods had sugar as either the most common or second most common ingredient; 55 percent contained artificial flavors; and 45 percent contained artificial colors.[21]

Symbolic of the hypocrisy of children's programming was the fare offered on one station on a Saturday morning (January 26, 1980 on CBS). At approximately 10:55, Popeye told the kids to brush and floss their teeth and to visit the dentist regularly. During the subsequent fifteen-minute period, the kids were exposed to a commercial for Lucky Charms cereal (sugar content=50.4 percent); Burger King (with a milk shake of carbohydrate content=68 percent); Post cereals, featuring a superheroes contest (on the average, half of the contents of the five advertised cereals—Super Sugar Crisp, Fruity Pebbles, Cocoa Pebbles, Alpha Bits, and Honeycombs—was sugar). Cookie Crisp cereal and the Star Trek promotion of a candy bar were the subjects of the remaining commercials.

Nutrition education starts in early childhood!

Advertising also increases the price of food. The cost of the ads run by food corporations is passed on to the consumer. The National Commission on Food Marketing found that retail prices of nationally advertised brands of many common foods average 20 percent higher than private label products of comparable quality.[22]

In testimony before the House Subcommittee on Monopolies and Commercial Law, Ralph Nader and Beverly Moore reported on studies that show that the power of advertising is so great that an increase in advertising expenditures is an order of magnitude more effective in increasing sales than a comparable decrease in prices.[23] So, in our much-vaunted food system, corporations are better off spending money for advertising and then increasing prices to pay for it than they are lowering prices. Advertising also increases food prices by promoting processed foods.

Those major national and multinational corporations that can afford large advertising expenditures are able to push smaller companies aside with refined advertising techniques. The wealthier companies are also given greater access to prime commercial time at cheaper rates than are companies that have less to spend on advertising. As mentioned earlier, the USDA reports that "competition in concentrated industries mainly occurs in terms of product variation, additional advertising, and promotion."[24] Again, proof that it is not the quality of the product or the efficiency of the large corporations that gives them their competitive advantage.

Advertising may also affect the worldview of our society. The constant exposure to manipulative messages may lead Americans to become cynical and distrustful. Who can gauge the effect on children of 20,000 presentations per year, on television alone, of messages that contain little true information, misused language, and manipulation? And the advertisers appear to have succeeded in their crusade to turn hunger and thirst into Nature's way of telling us to buy something. In the word of nutritionist Joan Gussow:

> The heavy advertising of beer and soft drinks, for example, delivers a message far more potent than the urging to buy any single product. In terms of this message, it doesn't really matter whether someone going to the refrigerator gets out a Pepsi or a Coke, a 7-Up or a Budweiser. What matters is that a thirsty American in the 1970s goes to the refrigerator to open up a container rather than the sink to open up the tap. That behavior has been sold to us.[25]

The Dairy Story I

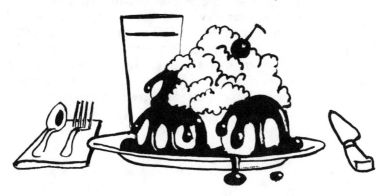

The National Dairy Council, an organization supported by contributions from dairy farmers and dairy processors, is one of the most important sources of nutrition education material in the country. The great resources of the NDC, and its tax-exempt status, allow it to provide attractive educational materials at low cost. Elementary school teachers in New York state reported that the Dairy Council is one of their three major sources of nutrition information.[1] In 1975, the Commissioners of Education in three states reported that Dairy Council representatives were in charge of teacher training in nutrition in those states.[2]

Why is the influence of the NDC on nutrition education a problem? Because the primary interest of the members of the Dairy Council is increasing the sales of dairy products, not in increasing our knowledge of nutrition.

An article by Eric Killburn in *Nutrition Action* points out the biases that appear in NDC nutrition education materials.[3] In "Little Ideas," a set of food pictures designed to help pre-schoolers identify foods, four of the sixteen milk products depicted are high in fat and two others are high in sugar. Of the eleven bread pictures, only one is of a whole grain product.

In "Food...Your Choice," elementary school children learn about the Four Basic Food Groups. They learn that ice cream and chocolate pudding belong in the healthful milk group, and that chocolate milk contains more protein than does skim milk. They do not learn that cheese is high in fat and moderately high in cholesterol. Little or no mention is made of dairy substitutes like margarine, or of food additives, or of junk foods, or of unfair advertising practices.

In "A Girl and Her Figure and You," teenagers learn that angel food cake and ice cream are low-calorie desserts, and in "Coronary Heart Disease: Risk Factors and the Diet Debate," the influence of diet on heart disease is downplayed and the saturated fat content of dairy products is ignored. An NDC memo on an early version of the Coronary Heart Disease pamphlet lists as one of its purposes, "to provide the dairy industry with a means to answer criticism aimed at dairy products, specifically milk-fat, in relation to heart disease." Fair enough, but not when disguised as an educational tool.

Education

Nutrition Quiz

1. What is choline? 2. What are the water-soluble vitamins? 3. On which vitamins is it easiest to overdose? 4. The caloric content of a gram of carbohydrate is (less than, equal to, greater than) the caloric content of a gram of fat. 5. True or False—In large enough doses all chemicals cause cancer. 6. Grains are a major source of which of the following? B vitamins, carbohydrate, fat, fiber, protein. 7. The use of oral contraceptives depletes bodily supplies of which nutrient?

Answers: 1. A B vitamin; 2. The vitamins which dissolve in water and, therefore, are excreted by the body, making overdose less likely. They include the B vitamins and vitamin C; 3. The vitamins that are fat soluble rather than water soluble, causing them to be stored in body fat rather than excreted, and making overdose more likely than is the case for the water soluble vitamins. They include Vitamins A, D, E, and K; 4. Less than; 5. False, only a small proportion of chemicals cause cancer in any dose; 6. All except fat; 7. Evidence is strongest for vitamin B6.

These questions deal with information that could be helpful to most people in planning a healthy diet. The questions do not call for sophisticated knowledge of the fine points of nutrition. Yet, while many Americans know where to go when "you deserve a break today" or how to get "tuna that tastes good, not tuna with good taste," most probably cannot answer these questions. In an FDA survey, only one-third of the homemakers who were interviewed reported that they know "quite a bit" about nutrition.[1] The small number of correct answers to the questions about nutrition included in the survey demonstrated the lack of nutrition knowledge of many Americans. One-quarter of the people answering did not know that fresh food is more nutritious than canned or frozen food; one-third did not know any of the nutrients in green peas; and less than half knew that milk is a source of vitamin D or that enriched bread is a source of carbohydrates.

Homemakers are not alone in their ignorance about nutrition. When public health nurses in British Columbia, Canada were given a nutrition quiz containing true or false question like "Potatoes and bread should be eliminated from the diet of someone trying to lose weight" (False) or "Green peppers, strawberries, and cantaloupes are good sources of Vitamin C" (True), the average score was 75 percent.[2] The poorest scores were achieved in the areas of nutritional requirements, the nutritional value of foods, the function of nutrients, and nutrition during pregnancy.

On another nutrition test, third and fourth year medical students and practicing physicians were able to answer only half of the questions correctly.[3] Whereas most of the doctors and medical students correctly identified a cholesterol-lowering diet, and almost all knew about the connection between obesity and diabetes mellitus, very few had heard of lactose intolerance, or correctly chose foods for a triglyceride-lowering diet, or knew what drugs interfere with the metabolism of folic acid (a B vitamin), and none of them knew which clinical conditions involve vitamin B6.

Finally, daycare teachers who took a nutrition knowledge test in 1976 correctly answered only slightly more than half of the questions.[4] So, part of the explanation for the ignorance about nutrition exhibited by most people is that nurses, teachers, and doctors, on whom we might rely for information, are themselves ignorant.

Another part of the explanation is suggested by a finding in the survey of daycare teachers. When asked what was their main source of information about nutrition, less than one out of ten of the teachers answered "school." Obviously nutrition education in schools is inadequate.

The inadequacy begins with the amount of nutrition education available in the schools. Teachers of kindergarten through sixth grade in New York state reported teaching an average of less than ten hours about nutrition and foods during 1974-75.[5] Even this small number is misleadingly large, for most of the nutrition education was given by a few of the teachers. One-quarter of the teachers did not teach any nutrition at all.

The unavailability of nutrition education continues right through medical school. In 1978, only one-quarter of the accredited medical schools in the United States offered a required course in nutrition, about half offered only elective courses, and one-fifth offered neither.[6] As a result, a survey of medical students found that fewer than one in five had taken a nutrition course either in college or in medical school.[7] In the words of Senator Patrick Leahy of Vermont, "There was far, far more time in the average medical school spent on the question of malpractice insurance...than there was on nutrition."[8]

The quality of nutrition education available in schools is also inadequate. Most teachers rely on the Four Basic Food Groups approach, which advises people to eat a combination of foods from a dairy group, a meat group, a fruit and vegetable group, and a grain group. Providing a scheme that simplifies nutrition education is probably a good idea, but the Basic Four approach is simplistic and out of date. The Basic Four treats skim milk and ice cream identically. It has no place for processed products like Twinkies and Cookie Crisp, except perhaps in the grain group, treated identically with whole wheat bread. The approach deals with avoiding deficiencies of nutrients, but not with the role food processing plays in this process, and ignores the problem of avoiding too much of substances like sugar, salt, fats, and additives.

Nutrition educators should teach people to feed themselves and their families cheaply and healthily, even when they are eating at a restaurant or have little time to prepare a meal. They should teach people how to prepare tasty meals from unprocessed foods like lentils or brown rice, and how to put together a healthy sandwich. At the present time they are failing at this task.

Biased Teaching Materials

One of the reasons for this failure is the quest of the food industry for profit. Even in the area of nutrition education in schools, agribusiness exerts a controlling influence. Many organizations representing the food industry, particularly the National Dairy Council, use low-cost educational materials to get their messages across. Often teachers are unaware of the corporate sponsorship and bias of these materials. For example, the film "Emphasis on Quality" is listed as being available from Association Films without listing the sponsorship of the Welch Foods Company.[9]

The materials are produced in the interest of the sponsors. A child learning about the Basic Four Food Groups from industry materials can discover that the dairy group includes Kellogg's cereal with milk, McDonalds thick shakes (which contain no whole milk), or Del Monte Pudding. Materials put out by Campbell, makers of soups with high salt contents, do not discuss the problems of excess salt intake. Those put out by Kelloggs, General Mills, or the Cereal Institute, ignore most of the problems resulting from excess sugar intake. The American Institute of Baking has put out a pamphlet claiming that "...leading nutritionists today accept enriched bread as being 'on par' with whole wheat bread."[10] And the National Soft Drink Association booklet "The Story of Soft Drinks" tells kids that "Water is another important ingredient of a balanced diet...we...need to drink 5-6 glasses a day. Soft drinks are about 90% purified water," but does not mention excessive sugar, calories, artificial colors, and other additives.[11]

Corporate sponsored materials are used in all areas of education, not just in nutrition education. As early as 1956, the Modern Talking Picture Service, specialists in business-subsidized distribution, was able to report that its films were being used by 26,000 clubs and youth groups, 36,000 churches, and 53,000 schools and colleges.[12]

The pamphlets, films, slide shows, and posters put out by industry are designed to promote consumption and/or to portray the activities of industry positively. In the words of a statement in *Printer's Ink,* a publication for marketing communications:

Eager minds can be molded to want your products: In the grade schools throughout America are nearly 23,000,000 young girls and boys. These children eat food, wear out clothes, use soap. They are consumers today and will be the buyers of tomorrow. Here is a vast market for your products. Sell these children on your brand name and they will insist that their parents buy no other.[13]

Sounds like the reasoning behind advertising to children doesn't it? And, just like advertising, if the materials were truly informative people might learn how to waste less, how to avoid being manipulated, and what not to buy. By now you do not have to be told how this would affect profits, and why, therefore, it may never come to pass.

There are noncorporate sources of material that can be used for real nutrition education. The Center for Science in the Public Interest (address listed in Appendix) puts out pamphlets, posters, books, and a very informative and easy to read newsletter called *Nutrition Action.* The bookstores listed in the Appendix will also sell you useful books and pamphlets by mail. The *Journal of Nutrition Education* often cites innovative methods and educational materials that can be helpful to teaching nutrition.

But the funds that are necessary to produce these materials and to make them available to schools at low cost are disproportionately controlled by industry. As a result, the corporate point of view is more likely than other viewpoints to be presented to students, under the guise of education, and therefore to be perceived by most people as the truth. Psychological studies have shown that people are more influenced by messages that they believe are meant to inform them than they are by messages that they believe are meant to influence them. The corporations hedge their bets by using both types. Think of the last McDonalds commercial you saw; then think of the last public relations spot put out by Mobil Oil on the wonders of free enterprise or on the horrors of government regulation; then think back to the films you saw in school on the miracle of the modern American farm, or on the dangers of insects, or on the road travelled by bananas from the plantation to your table. These are all forms of corporate propaganda, ranging from the obvious to the subtle.

The educational system influences our eating not only directly, by teaching (or not teaching) us about food and nutrition, but also indirectly by molding our view of the world. Which socioeconomic systems are good and which are bad? What has happened in the past and, therefore, what changes might be possible in the future? The answers that we give to these questions are greatly influenced by what we learn in school and, in turn, influence the kind of society, including the food system, that we believe in.

As in many societies, the American educational system primarily propogates the official view of reality. We learn, in social studies, how a bill becomes a law in a democracy, but not how much influence industry has over the process. We are taught a view of history that depicts American free enterprise as the source of much of the world's recent social progress and that portrays U.S. foreign policy as simply the defense of freedom. In learning about the causes of World War I, were you told that the Lusitania, the British liner with American passengers aboard that was sunk by a German submarine, carried large amounts of ammunition sent from the U.S. to Great Britain in order to kill German soldiers? When you learned about the Pullman strike that was ended when President Cleveland dispatched troops, did you learn why the workers were striking? Did you learn about the Nonpartisan League, which earlier in this century elected the Governor of North Dakota and instituted such "socialist" practices as a state bank that made credit more easily available to small farmers?

The lessons taught in schools can provide tools that allow people to think for themselves and to overcome manipulation. They can also provide opportunities for that manipulation. To date, the American educational system has provided the tools of literacy and some minimal access to opposing viewpoints to many people. But has also reinforced a viewpoint slanted in favor of American business and, thus, failed to teach people the fundamentals of good nutrition.

The Saccharin Story

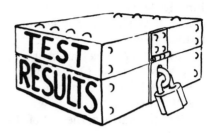

The studies that demonstrated that saccharin probably causes cancer, and that led to a proposed ban on the drug in March 1977, created an uproar. In 1976, about seven million pounds of saccharin were used in foods—10 percent in table top artificial sweeteners like Sweet 'n Low, 15 percent in dietetic foods, and 75 percent in diet soda pop. The companies that made big money from selling saccharin or products made with saccharin sponsored a public relations campaign designed to discredit the studies. Frequently mentioned criticisms of the studies included the use of rats as subjects and the use of test doses on the rats that were equivalent to a massive intake of saccharin by humans—sometimes as much as 800 cans of diet soda pop a day, with the implication that in large enough doses almost any substance would cause cancer.

The scientific criticism of the use of rats is silly. If animals are not used as test subjects, then humans would have to be used. It is sometimes possible to measure the effects on humans of ingesting a substance that has been on the market for a while, but these tests have a number of weaknesses. First, outside of the laboratory, people ingest many substances. Those people who use saccharin are probably also more likely to ingest other substances associated with dieting, such as grapefruit, diet pills, and cottage cheese. Thus, studies done outside of the controlled conditions of the laboratory are less able to link a health hazard like cancer to the ingestion of one particular substance like saccharin. Second, cancer often takes decades to develop and widespread use of saccharin only began in the 1960s, so not enough time has elapsed to allow scientists to measure the full carcinogenic (cancer causing) effect of the drug. The use of test animals allows scientists to draw conclusions about the safety of a substance before thousands of people have been made ill. Of course, there is no guarantee that rats will react the same as humans, but in the past many species have shown a general similarity in their response to carcinogens. Finally, some studies of humans that have contracted bladder cancer have shown a connection to saccharin intake. Nonetheless, industry scientists continue to criticize the use of animal tests, sometimes reaching the absurdity of the medical director of Exxon, who wrote in the *Cancer Bulletin* that "When a carcinogen is prevented from entering the environment on the basis of screening results, there can be no data regarding that exposure in man."

On the surface, the use of the large doses seems to be a more important weakness of the studies. After all, nobody drinks 800 cans of diet soda pop a day, so why the big fuss? Large doses are used because a particular cancer strikes only a small proportion of people. Lung cancer, for example, occurs in only about one out of every 2,500 people. But, with an American population of 220 million, even a substance that caused cancer in only one out 10,000 people would affect 22,000 Americans and would thus be very dangerous. Testing the carcinogenic effects of such a substance using normal doses, however, would not be easy because fifty or sixty thousand test animals would be needed in order to have the cancer appear in just a few of the exposed animals. As the use of such a large number of animals is impractical, scientists use a smaller number of animals and give each animal a larger than normal dose of the substance being tested. Thus, instead of thirty million Americans ingesting the saccharin in two to four cans of diet soda pop for thirty years, one hundred rats ingest the equivalent of hundreds of cans a day for one year. The scientists must assume that the large doses used in the study make up for the short duration and the small number of subjects. Most substances tested in this manner, even using large quantities, do not cause cancer. And saccharin has been found to be carcinogenic in quantities equivalent to as little as one and a half cans of diet soda pop a day.

The tests are obviously not perfect, but they are the best sources of information about the health hazards produced by saccharin. It would be insane to use millions of test animals or to wait for cancer to develop in thousands of people before taking action, no matter what the medical director of Exxon thinks. The use of animals as test subjects and of high doses to make up for the limited number of these subjects is based on assumptions that have worked in the past. The corporate critics of the studies do not provide any practical alternatives to them. The Calorie Control Council, an industry organization, has repeatedly attacked the Canadian study that led to the proposed ban even though the council was shown the study while it was being planned and returned the plan without comment. But profit is an important inducement, so despite the twenty-three studies in the 1970s that found a link between saccharin and cancer, and the lack of studies finding that saccharin helps people to lose weight, and the fact that one out of five American deaths is due to cancer, industry spokespeople continue their propaganda against the studies.

Based on information taken from Samuel S. Epstein, *The Politics of Cancer*. Garden City: Anchor, 1979, pp. 1, 11, 38, 57, 191-199

Health

Germs surround us. Bacteria follow us wherever we go. Our best friends transmit viruses. Every day our bodies are host to thousands of these disease-producing organisms. So why aren't we sick all of the time? Because humans, like most other species, have developed mechanisms that allow us to resist the pathogens that cause disease. In the words of one writer, "Health...does not mean the absence of disturbances but rather an effective bodily reaction toward them..."[1]

If they are functioning properly, the resistance mechanisms will keep us in good health. When illness does occur, the mechanisms will usually fight it off in a short time. So the key to good health would seem to be to avoid being overwhelmed by pathogens and to keep the resistance mechanisms functioning properly. At times it may be necessary to go further and give the resistance mechanisms a helping hand with drugs or surgery, but that should be a last resort.

Unfortunately, in this society these priorities are reversed. Publicity, prestige, and financial support go primarily to medicine, which relies on drugs and surgery, rather than to public health, which controls the spread of pathogens, or prevention, which maintains the resistance mechanisms. A new transplant operation makes headlines. Physicians are paid outlandish sums. Being a doctor accords far more social status than being a nutritionist or a public health specialist. So much stress is put on fancy techniques for curing disease that drugs are often over-prescribed and surgery is sometimes needlessly done. According to the Committee on Interstate and Foreign Commerce of the U.S. House of Representatives, in 1973, American surgeons performed over three million unnecessary operations that cost nearly $5 billion, and killed about 16,000 patients.[2]

This system makes little sense. Of course, medical procedures are sometimes necessary, but it is usually more efficient to prevent problems from developing than to try to deal with the problems one at a time after they develop. Public health and preventive measures are cheaper and help more people than do medical techniques. And, despite beliefs to the contrary, these measures have been more effective than medicine in the fight against disease. According to a recent book:

> Tuberculosis, for instance, reached a peak over two generations. In New York in 1812, the death rate was estimated to be higher than 700 per 10,000; by 1882, when Koch first isolated and cultured the bacillus, it had already declined to 370 per 10,000. The rate was down to 180 when the first sanatorium was opened in 1910, even though "consumption" still held second place in the mortality tables. After World War II, but before antibiotics became routine, it had slipped into eleventh place with a rate of forty-eight. Cholera, dysentery, and typhoid similarly peaked and dwindled outside the physicians control. By the time their etiology [cause] was understood and their therapy had become specific, these diseases had lost much of their virulence and hence their social importance. The combined death rate from scarlet fever, diphtheria, whooping cough, and measles among children up to fifteen shows that nearly 90 percent of the total decline in mortality between 1860 and 1965 had occurred before the introduction of antibiotics and widespread immunization.[3]

Improved sanitation, clean water, good food, and decent housing have done more to keep people healthy than tricky surgery, fancy drugs, and expensive technology.

Attention to food and nutrition is a measure of both public health and prevention. Pathogens that spread infectious diseases and chemicals that cause cancer and birth defects may be contained in food. And good nutrition supplies the energy and the raw materials that are needed for the optimal functioning of the body's natural resistance mechanisms. Yet, the health establishment still pays much less attention to nutrition than to drugs or surgery.

When was the last time that your doctor asked you to detail exactly what you have been eating or measured the nutrients in your blood and hair? If you are like most people, probably never. As the surveys in chapter 7 show, most doctors wouldn't even know what to do with information about nutrition if they did collect it.

In fact, doctors may actually add to the level of poor nutrition in America. The do this by prescribing drugs without attending to the nutritional effects of the drug usage and by paying little attention to the food served in hospitals. A number of studies have shown that nutrition in hospitals is not very good. One study even found that many people who are adequately nourished upon entering the hospital show signs of malnutrition after spending a few weeks there.[4]

Why Is Nutrition Downplayed?

Doctors pay little attention to nutrition for several reasons. In addition to poor medical education, there is the attitude that every problem has a technological solution. According to this notion, if we look hard enough we will find a chemical, a machine, or a technique to cure every ailment. Related to this attitude is the overspecialization that occurs throughout our society. In medicine this takes the form of doctors who are experts in certain parts of the body but who do not deal with other parts, when even most lay people realize that the different parts affect one another. The overspecialization can become so extreme that several doctors may simultaneously treat the same patient without being fully aware of the treatments being used or the drugs being prescribed by their colleagues. Also, the aura of technical expertise surrounding modern medicine places doctors in positions of prestige and power vis-a-vis their patients. This power would be greatly reduced if health care focused more on preventive measures that could be practiced by non-experts.

But there is a more important reason that prevention, in general and nutrition, in particular, are not stressed in our health care system. Imagine a society where the consumption of fresh food is promoted and the consumption of junk food is discouraged; where chemicals are used to grow crops, raise animals, and process food only when absolutely necessary; where people are taught the fundamentals of good nutrition and are given time to prepare healthy meals; where the pollution of the earth, air, and sea is tightly controlled; where everyone has access to decent health care, but drugs and surgery are used only as a last resort; where hospitalization is discouraged but is made available at low cost when it is truly needed.

This society would be a healthy one but it would be missing the giant profits so important to some. A society that stresses prevention, public health, and nutrition, rather than medicine, surgery, and hospitalization is less profitable to the food industry that relies on processing, junk foods, and overconsumption, to the industries that pollute the environment, to the hospital, pharmaceutical, and medical equipment industries, and to the doctors who get rich attempting to cure our ailments. Rather than lose profits to promote health by being more careful about the products it produces and the methods it uses to produce those products, industry is able to market health, and thus increase profits, by selling us lots of expensive drugs, equipment, and expertise.

The ancient Greeks believed that illness signified a lack of balance between a person and the universe. Being modern, we scoff at such primitive, unscientific ideas. But our economic system is unbalanced in that most people have little say over what is produced and how it is produced. These decisions are based almost entirely upon private profit, largely ignoring social, cultural, environmental, and health concerns, causing further imbalance. The chapters of this book illustrate the many ways in which these imbalances affect the diet of everyone who is a member of our society. It may be fair to conclude that our unbalanced diets result from an unbalanced socioeconomic system. The Greeks were right: our illnesses do signify a lack of balance between us and the universe.

As a result of this unbalanced system U.S. health costs have increased eightfold over the last two decades, far outstripping the overall inflation rate, while the average income of doctors is over $61,000.[5] The United States certainly has better health care than many poor nations, but it is the only advanced industrial nation in the world not to have a national health care system, and in 1977 it only ranked thirteenth in the world in infant mortality, with the proportion of children dying before their first birthday being almost twice as high in the U.S. as in Sweden.[6]

The poorest people, of course, suffer the most from American health problems. In a 1977 survey conducted by the Department of Health, Education and Welfare, only 5 percent of people from families with an income of $25,000 or more reported that their health was fair or poor, compared to 24 percent of people from families with an income of less than $5,000.[7] Blacks die of heart diseases and cancer at a rate that is a third again as high as that of whites, and the mortality from diabetes of blacks is over twice as high as that of whites.[8]

Nationwide studies of nutritional intake find that many Americans may be suffering from nutritional deficiencies. For example, the Health and Nutrition survey of the United States, conducted by the Department of Health, Education and Welfare between 1971 and 1974, found that about one-third of white male ten and eleven year olds received from their diets less than the standards set by the government for vitamin C intake.[9] Two-thirds of females aged 65 and over were below the standard set for iron intake. Half of the four and five year olds were below the niacin (vitamin B3) standard. And three-quarters of poor black males aged twenty-five to thirty-four received inadequate levels of vitamin A from their food. Even if surveys such as this one overestimate somewhat the level of nutritional deficiencies, as some experts believe, they indicate that many Americans may be deficient in some important nutrients at the same time that they are consuming too much of other nutrients.

Dietary problems have been linked to six of the ten leading causes of death in the United States.[10] The rate of coronary heart disease has been related to the excess intake of saturated fat and cholesterol. It has also been linked to the overconsumption of salt (which promotes high blood pressure) and, in some studies, to the overconsumption of sugar and the underconsumption of fiber. The rate of stroke may also be related to salt consumption in that salt intake increases blood pressure which increases the likelihood of stroke. The rate of arteriosclerosis has been connected to fat consumption, and cirrhosis of the liver is certainly related to alcohol intake. Diabetes occurs much more often in people who are obese than in non-obese people and has been linked, in some studies, to the consumption of too much sugar and too little fiber. Some studies indicate that the intake of fat may be a factor in causing certain cancers.

Based on these relationships, the Senate Select Committee on Nutrition and Human Needs released a set of dietary goals in 1977.[11] The goals suggested that: about half of the calories in our diet should come from the complex carbohydrates and naturally occurring sugars found in fruits, vegetables, and whole grains; only one-tenth of the calories should come from refined and processed sugars; total fat consumption should account for less than one-third of the calories, and of that 30 percent, saturated fats should only account for a third (totaling 10 percent of the overall diet); and, cholesterol and salt consumption should be limited.

Food industry experts dispute most studies that link diet and disease. They point out the problems of each study. But as the saccharin story demonstrates, the connection between environmental factors and disease is never easy to make. Each type of study has its own weakness. As a result, we can either listen to the food industry and ignore all of the imperfect studies (the tobacco industry still discounts the overwhelming evidence linking cigarette smoking and cancer) or we can base our personal and policy decisions regarding health and diet on the best evidence that is available.

This does not mean that we must all become health food freaks. Although many foods marketed as health foods are excellent, some foods sold in the name of health are not. Many of the brands of vitamins for children that come in the shape of cartoon characters contain sugar and are missing some important nutrients. Some commercial health food cereals and many of the snacks sold in health food stores contain large amounts of honey or brown sugar. While these health food sweeteners sometimes contain more nutrients than does regular sugar, they are only marginally better for you. So, although a sweet snack here and there is not really bad for you, don't think that you can get away with anything by frequently satisfying your sweet tooth with health food cakes and candies.

Some nutrition experts get a little carried away with the role played by bad eating in our society. They claim, for example, that excess intake of sugar is responsible for everything from the rising American divorce rate to the Holocaust. In the future we will probably find that improved nutrition can help us to deal with many problems that have not previously been connected to eating. But we cannot just assume these connections, we must prove them.

Many psychological problems have been linked to poor nutrition in good scientific research done at the University of Minnesota in the 1950s and at the Massachusetts Institute of Technology at the present time. If resources are made available for good research, important discoveries will be made about correct eating and about the effects of poor nutrition, but only if those resources are not controlled by physicians who are ignorant about nutrition and who do not believe that it is worth studying, or by representatives of the food industry who want to protect the profits to be made from selling devitalized, highly processed food.

In the meantime, you would do well to do some research of your own. If you read or hear about a claim that changing your eating—eliminating some food from your diet or taking a vitamin or mineral supplement—will help you in some way, pay serious attention to it, but check out the evidence used to support the claim. Were any studies done? How many people have been helped so far? What kind of people; old, young, well, sick? Can the change harm you in any way? If you decide to try to make a change, carefully observe your reaction. How do you feel before the change? How do you feel after? If there is an improvement, does it last? After a while go back to your old way of eating for a short time. Does the improvement disappear? If the new way of eating causes a lasting marked improvement that disappears when you go back to the old way, then you are on to something.

Amateur research like this is obviously not useful for answering such questions as does increased intake of selenium reduce susceptiblilty to cancer. In the long run, the best answer to nutritional problems will be to change our health care and food systems. But an open minded yet skeptical person can learn to treat many day-to-day health problems with good nutrition and careful use of nutritional supplements by reading such sources as *Prevention Magazine, Executive Health,* and the *Newsletter of the International Academy of Preventive Medicine.* Skin problems, migraine headaches, and fatigue, as well as more serious illnesses such as diabetes, have been successfully treated with dietary changes. A growing number of doctors and other health specialists are stressing prevention. (To find out the names and addresses of many of these people you can write to the International Academy of Preventive Medicine. See Appendix for the address.) The United States has the resources to become one of the healthiest societies in history. Right now those resources are being used to increase profits rather than health. But we can change that situation.

The Soda Pop Story

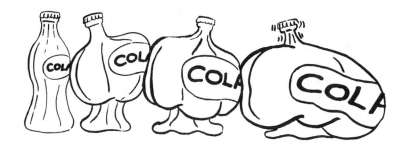

In 1849, Americans consumed less than two eight-ounce servings of soda pop per person.[1] By 1909, twenty-three years after the invention of Coca Cola, we were drinking sixteen eight-ounce servings per person. Forty years later consumption had risen tenfold. Twenty years after that, it doubled again, reaching the incredible figure of 574 eight-ounce servings of soft drinks per person in 1978. But these are just the average figures. According to government surveys, one out of five American adults (eighteen to forty-four years old) drinks at least two soft drinks a day.[2] Soft drinks account for about one-quarter of total American sucrose (table sugar) consumption, a whopping 23.2 pounds per person each year.[3] If we multiply the 439 eight-ounce servings of non-diet soft drinks consumed by the average American in 1976 by the twelve calories per ounce in Coke, 7-Up, or Dr. Pepper, we find that in that year the average American consumed 42,144 calories in the form of soft drinks. Dividing that figure by the approximately 3,500 calories that produce a pound of body weight, we find that soft drinks accounted for twelve pounds on the average American in 1976. Just for fun, we can multiply this figure by the approximate American population of 200 million to determine that soft drinks accounted for about 2.5 *billion* pounds of American weight in 1976.

The folks in the beverage industry eventually realized the effect they were having on the American waistline and, being good citizens, they decided to do something about it. They might have cut down on their promotion (Coca Cola spent $184.2 million on advertising in 1980[4]) and advised people to go back to cheap, thirst-quenching water, but of course that would have decreased profits.

Instead they developed another great American innovation—the diet soft drink. That way they could "help" overweight people and themselves at the same time. In 1976, the average American drank about fifty-four eight-ounce servings of artificially sweetened soft drinks.[5] Approximately one out of ten white American females (ages eighteen to forty-four) drinks at least one artifically sweetened drink a day.[6] (Figures for males and for black females are slightly lower.) So now the beverage industry has the honor of being a major purveyor of carcinogenic saccharine (see chapter 8) as well as a sugar pusher.

Eating Disorders

Jane is 18 years old. Her parents are well off and she has always been an obedient daughter and a good student. Slightly "plump" as a child, Jane began a diet soon after going away to college. The diet never stopped. When her weight went down to 80 pounds, Jane's parents took her out of school and had her hospitalized. She would talk endlessly about food and would spend hours shopping and cooking, but she never ate more than a few mouthfuls.

Sarah is a 23-year-old assistant buyer for a department store. She is not slim, but she is far from being obese. On weekends, Sarah binges on whole pizza pies, bags of taco chips, and gallons of ice cream. After each binge, she walks into her bathroom, sticks her fingers down her throat, and throws up. Later, she takes a few large swigs from the laxative bottle that she keeps in her medicine cabinet. She has been repeating this routine for two and a half years, but she is embarrassed to tell anyone about it.

Francine is a 42-year-old homemaker. She put on a few extra pounds when she had her daughter and went on a diet that she read about in a magazine. Since that time, she has been on many diets, purchased many products designed to firm up various parts of her body, and joined many different organizations in an attempt to keep her weight down. She never weighs more than about 15 pounds over what she considers to be her ideal weight, but she also never stops thinking about her weight or loses that feeling of restraining herself around food.

Bill is a 50-year-old history teacher. He has a fondness for pasta and beer. In high school, he was on the basketball team and he was in very good shape. Since then, however, he has not been very active physically. After work, he reads or watches televsion and on weekends he goes to a ballgame or to the movies. Although he is not greatly overweight, he does sport an impressive pot belly.

The cases of Jane, Sarah, Francine, and Bill exemplify some of the weight and eating problems prevalent in the United States today. Although these cases are fictional, they each depict behaviors that are typical of many thousands of people. What causes so many Americans to suffer from eating disorders and weight problems?

Fat and Females

Part of the answer to this question undoubtedly has something to do with the gender of the people suffering from these problems. It was no accident that I described the cases of three women and one man, for not only do studies show that a greater proportion of women than men are overweight,[1] but other problems associated with food appear to be nearly exclusive to women. The membership of reducing organizations are almost entirely composed of women.[2] Anorexics, like Jane, who intentionally starve themselves, and bulimarexics, like Sarah, who purge themselves after bingeing, are also overwhelmingly female.[3] Although many men in our society are concerned with watching their waistlines, with cutting fats and calories to maintain youthful proportions and healthy bodies, the problems surrounding weight and eating have never reached the level among boys and men that they have among girls and women. The extent of these problems among women is perhaps most strongly demonstrated by a government survey that found that half of the women in the U.S. consider themselves to be overweight.[4]

In order to understand these problems, we have to look beyond individual weaknesses of character or mere failures of willpower to the position of women in contemporary American society—to cultural images and social roles and how they have been changing. Although gender-linked weight problems appear to be relatively recent phenomena, the mistreatment of women's bodies in order to bring them closer to the standard of beauty current in a particular society has been going on for many years. Before the 1948 revolution, the feet of many girls in traditional Chinese society were bound because women with tiny feet were considered to be attractive. As depicted in the movie *Gone with the Wind*, many nineteenth century American women had to wear excruciatingly tight corsets and unwieldy bustles in order to present the hourglass figure demanded of them.

And when the fashions changed, the women were supposed to change. To attain the milk-white complexion fashionable in upper-class British society in the 1820s and 1830s, women were told to stay out of the sun, to eat potatoes, and to avoid all other vegetables, butter, milk, cheese, cream, and fish. (The parallel is disgusting, but how different is this from the treatment given to the calves bred for veal described in chapter 1?) Today, women are told to spread cocoa butter or banana oil on their skins and bake in the sun in order to attain a "San Tropez" tan. (Many of these standards of beauty are impossible for non-white women to attain.)

Similar changes have occurred in the American standard of the proper proportions of women's bodies. When the plump image of Lillian Russell and Lily Langtry, the "sex symbols" of the Gay Nineties, gave way to the ideal of the skinny, boyish flapper of the Roaring Twenties, the eroticism of the fleshy figure became devalued. The rounded thighs, arms, and bellies idealized in Western art since the Renaissance and epitomized by Rubens were discarded. Studies show that in the recent past the standards of thinness have become even more stringent. Over the past two decades, for example, Playboy centerfolds and winners of the Miss America contest have become increasingly thin.[5]

Wherever women look they get the message that slim is in. A study of magazines found that the most popular women's magazine in 1980 contained seventeen times as many articles and advertisements dealing with body weight and dieting as did the most poplular men's magazines.[6] A study of the top forty television shows in March 1982 found that of the male characters appearing on the shows, less than one-fifth were slim and more than one-quarter were plump, whereas of the female characters, over two-thirds were slim and only one-tenth were plump.[7] In addition, medical doctors will sometimes communicate their feelings to patients that slim is healthy despite recent studies that find that, at least among women, only those people that are extremely overweight or underweight risk early death.[8]

A particularly obnoxious role in promoting the slim standard is played by advertisers. Remember, advertisers are happiest when they can create unfillable needs. Satisfaction and self-acceptance are bad business to them. They know that adult women will never look like adolescents. There is no reason why they should. But in convincing the public that a teenager such as Brooke Shields is the acme of feminine attractiveness and in selecting models from among a small number of children and anorexic adults, advertisers set a standard that most women can never reach. That keeps women constantly dissatisfied (hence the finding that 50 percent of American women considered themselves to be overweight), constantly striving to fix themselves, and thus constantly buying— clothes, cosmetics, depilatories, and diet products.

The role played by husbands, boyfriends, and fathers in promoting the obsession with slimness is not yet fully understood.

On the one hand, these men often reinforce the notion that women are judged based upon their bodies. On the other hand, many men say that they prefer women with fleshy breasts, behinds, and thighs, an attitude that is no less body-oriented than the Brooke Shields ideal, but that nonetheless should be expected, if men's standards were simply pushed upon women, to counter the pressure to be slim.

The standards are backed up by emotions. A series of studies demonstrated that fat people are rated as less likable than people who are lame, missing limbs, or facially deformed.[9] These factors play a role in causing the chronic dieting and obsession with weight of many American women.

This is not to say, however, that obesity and overeating are never problems in and of themselves. Many Americans are out of shape and a large number may be compulsive eaters or may frequently "pig out" on junk food. While it is a great error to apply an overly stringent standard of slimness, it is also an error to ignore the food abuse and eating disorders that are now prevalent in the United States.

Here again the problem is particularly bad for women, for not only are they supposed to be slim sex objects, they are also supposed to be nurturing—providing a soft shoulder to cry on, a clean, comfortable home to live in, and healthy, tasty meals to eat. Traditionally, women and men shared the food-provider role. But in industrial, consumer society, the food that most people eat is bought and prepared by women. Women spend more time than do men in supermarkets and kitchens. When they are not surrounded by the real thing, women are confronted with images of food. The same study that found that the most popular women's magazines contain more articles and ads relating to dieting and weight than do the most popular men's magazines also found that women's magazines contain seventy times the number of food-related articles and ads as do the men's magazines.[10] Thus, women are first surrounded by food and told to spend a great deal of time thinking about and preparing it, and then they are expected to undergo all sorts of dietary contortions to attain "ideal" proportions. Is it any wonder that many women become fanatic dieters while many others become compulsive eaters?

Lifestyle

Yet many men do have problems with food and weight, for eating disorders are caused by more than sexism. As discussed in chapter 5, our society is undergoing an economic and social transformation that has affected sex roles, family structure, and the composition of the workforce. Due to the increasing participation of women in the labor force, the number of households in which one or more members is free to plan, shop for, and prepare meals on a full-time basis is steadily diminishing. This leaves many men with the responsibility for preparing their own food, sharing the preparation with their living partners, or suffering the consequences of relying on commercial food preparation.

Our eating habits are obviously affected by more than just the food industry. Modern urban life puts pressure on our eating too. Many of us wake up each morning in time to wash, dress, grab a quick bite, then hit the rush-hour commute to work. The balanced breakfast recommended by nutritionists is impractical for people on tight schedules. Few people work close enough to home to return for a substantial, healthful lunch, so most of us rely on delis, fast-food restaurants, or cafeterias, perhaps squeezing lunch into a quick break between errands. Often it is easiest to buy coffee-break snacks from a cart or vending machine. Dinner must often be prepared by a hungry person just returned home from a full workday, who may be too tired to exert even the minimal effort required to make a salad, steam some vegetables, and broil some fish.

So fat is due, in part, to a lifestyle which does not result from personal choice. Forty-hour work weeks, commuting, nuclear families, communities designed for cars rather than for legs are all aspects of our society that have evolved since the last century and that are beyond the control of individuals. When experts say that Americans are fat because they "choose" a fat lifestyle, they are ignoring the social forces that affect that lifestyle. While, as a group, Americans must take responsibilty for improving the system under which we live, individual Americans should not be blamed for the consequences built into modern life over which we have little control.

Effects of the AFS

Psychologist Stanley Schachter has shown that many people, especially overweight people, rely on external cues to determine when and what they eat.[11] Instead of relying on internal cues, like physical sensations of hunger, these people respond to the sight or smell of food, or even to the time of day.

External food cues begin with bottle-feeding schedules. Many Americans grow up hearing the lunch-hour bell in school, then we have scheduled lunch hours on the job. Even the messages of advertising affect when and what we eat. Naomi Aronson points out that in a system where creating demand is a primary aim, it is not surprising that people eat on the basis of external cues to satisfy demands other than the purely nutritional.[12]

In earlier chapters we saw how food marketing and advertising are designed to create or exaggerate needs for food products in order to maximize sales. We also saw how the physiological mechanisms regulating hunger and satiety represent a natural limitation that must be overcome to maximize profits. To this end, the industry promotes snacking so that consumers will have more than three opportunities a day to consume food, replaces free water with purchased soft drinks, presents desserts as the ultimate reward, and bombards women and children with artificially glamorized images of highly processed foods.

We have also seen how the food industry appears to be having a love affair with sugar. The ads extol sweetness and frequently focus on highly sugared foods, especially when the ads are aimed at kids. Food labels are designed to disguise the excessive levels of sweeteners in many products by listing them separately (e.g. as dextrose, sucrose, corn syrup, sorbitol).

Food processors add sugar to nearly everything, from Campbell's Tomato Soup to Heinz Baked Beans. In so doing, they claim that they are giving consumers what we want. But, as with many other rationalizations, this one has only a small basis in truth. Sure, many of us crave sweets. During early human evolution, sweet tastes probably signaled edible fruit high in some nutrients. The desire for sweetness would then have had some survival value for humans and may have become "wired" into our nervous systems.

But human behavior can never be explained simply as instinctive. We are the products of the complex interaction of inborn tendencies with experience. Our genetic foundation may set limits on our learning experiences, but it does not exclusively determine our behavior. To understand the behavior of a rapist, we would not point to his desire for sex; we would try to understand how that desire became distorted by social and environmental factors, turning the act of sex into an act of violence. Similarly, to understand the modern American fondness for sweets, it is not enough to point to an inherent desire for sugar, even if scientists conclusively proved that such a desire exists; we must also understand how the food industry plays upon this desire to achieve its own ends. Americans don't ask to have sugar put into soup or to have our children constantly exposed to ads promoting sugary products. Whatever our inherent craving for sweets, the food industry exacerbates it with subtle additives as well as blatant advertising campaigns.

Sweets are only one source of concentrated calories. Another major source of calories heavily promoted by the food industry is processed foods. Of course, not every processed food contains more calories than its fresh counterpart, but many do. And prepared meals, such as tv dinners, often heap together a fattening combination of foods that a home meal planner might avoid, like breaded chicken with mashed potatoes, starchy peas, and syrup-packed fruit. A half cup of Del Monte canned French green beans has one and a half times as many calories as a similar portion of fresh green beans; an ear of Birds Eye frozen corn on the cob has almost twice the calories of an ear of fresh corn; a half cup of Libby's canned peach halves has almost three times the calories of a fresh two-inch peach.[13]

The other ways that the food industry promotes obesity are less well researched and so remain somewhat speculative. Dr. Theodore van Itallie, head of the first nationally funded obesity research center at St. Lukes Hospital in New York City, has suggested that fiber, which promotes chewing and satiety, may also inhibit fat storage and overeating.[14] The lack of fiber in many processed foods may thus contribute to obesity. Processing also depletes many trace minerals and other nutrients from our foods, altering their nutritional balance. Such imbalances may hinder the way we metabolize food. For example, unrefined grains contain complex carbohydrates and B vitamins. Proper digestion of the carbohydrates depends on the way these B vitamins work together. But, as discussed in the Bread Story, these vitamins are largely destroyed in the process of refining. Some of these vitamins are replaced with synthetic versions, but only some of them, and these are replaced at unnaturally high levels.

As if this weren't bad enough, the carbohydrate content of the refined grains is often increased during processing by the addition of sugar. The resulting imbalances of B vitamins with one another, and with the carbohydrates, may lead to an underutilization of nutrients, and the excess carbohydrates may be stored as fat.

Nutrient imbalances in the American diet may also underlie some food cravings and overeating. Lab animals raised on diets lacking particular nutrients often develop cravings for foods containing those nutrients. Malnourished people have also been known to eat clay or laundry starch to obtain the minerals lacking in their diets. It is possible that some of our food cravings stem from this sort of nutrient deprivation, so that even when we eat in quantity, we experience only a low level of satisfaction.

Another possible cause of overeating may reside in the high sugar content of our foods. Some researchers have claimed that the high levels of sugar in the American diet lead to hypoglycemia. Here's a simplified explanation of what that means: Sugar (glucose) is a simple carbohydrate, unlike the complex carbohydrates found in fruits, vegetables, cereals, or grains. When carbohydrates are eaten, the pancreas secretes insulin to help digest them. Simple sugars, which break down faster than complex carbohydrates, also enter the bloodstream much faster. When sugar is a frequent part of the diet, the pancreas may become sensitized to it. The pancreas then secretes massive quantities of insulin whenever sugar in ingested in order to reduce the high sugar content in the blood. The insulin levels may become so high that your glucose level may fall too low—even below fasting levels. When blood sugar levels become too low, many people report feelings of fatigue, irritability, poor concentration, and hunger, especially a craving for sweets. Hypoglycemics may fall prey to a vicious cycle in which high insulin levels knock blood sugar levels low enough to set off sweets craving; satisfying the craving raises the blood sugar high enough to overstimulate the pancreas, and so on. The portrait of a hypoglycemic is a person who can't seem to control sweets cravings, who therefore puts on too much weight, and who constantly feels listless and irritable.

While the evidence presented in earlier chapters implicating the food industry in causing nutrient imbalance and excessive intake of simple sugars is strong, the ways in which these mechanisms may lead to overeating are as yet only imperfectly understood.

One conclusion is clear: we live in a society in which food is produced for profit. The more we think about food and the more food we eat, the easier it is for those who control our food supply to acquire profit. Obsessions with weight and overeating are consonant with American enterprise; the food industry profits from our weight gains. But it also gains from our weight losses! A large diet industry has developed that reaps massive profits from people who yo-yo in weight.

The Diet Industry

Most accounts of the diet industry put its yearly sales at $10 billion.[15] The number and variety of diets available is astounding. In the name of weight loss, we can choose to count calories and ignore carbohydrates, or do just the reverse. We can drink seven glasses of water a day or continue to imbibe alcohol. We can gorge on grapefruits, eggs, bananas, even on ice cream. We can peel the skin from our chicken, eliminate the corn starch from our chop suey, or the flour from our bread. Some books promise we can eat anything we want and still lose weight.

Nearly every food seems to have a dietetic version. Fruits and vegetables are diet packed; salad dressings are made in oil-free versions. There are even diet cookies and candies. Pharmacies are stocked with pills, potions, powders, and capsules designed to rid us of that dreaded drive—appetite. These nostrums with medical-sounding names like Prolamine, Bioslim T, or Dietrix consist mainly of caffeine and fillers like cellulose. Another aisle in the same drugstore might proffer exercycles, reducing belts, or nylon sweatsuits for those who wish to lose water weight if they cannot lose fat.

If these don't work, someone is always happy to help—for a price. We can consult M.D.s, therapists, hypnotists, hospitals, clinics, and for the wealthy, fat farms and spas. We can join groups where we admit to being compulsive eaters and others that train us to ignore being overweight.

Then there are the last-resort techniques that force us to reduce despite ourselves. We can have our jaws wired, our intestines re-routed, our fat surgically scooped out. The miracle diets and cures at best allow us to lose a few pounds a week. At worst, they are completely ineffectual and unhealthful. By June of 1978, for example, fifty-eight deaths associated with very low calorie liquid protein diets had been reported, sixteen of them among women aged twenty-three to fifty-one who had no underlying medical problems that could have contributed to the deaths.[16]

Ironically, many of the companies that produce the products that help us to lose weight also produce those that help us put it on in the first place. The Soda Pop Story provides one obvious example. Louis Sherry, which offers us sugarless jams, produces rich, sugary ice cream. H.J. Heinz, the maker of 200 (not just 57 varieties) of foods—including La Pizzeria pizza and Mrs. Good-cookies—is also the owner of Weight Watchers, which in 1980 had half a million members.[17] Heinz acquired the weight-loss organization in 1978 for a hefty $71 million. It would appear that big waistlines mean big profits, and that in the unlikely event that we all permanently attained our desired weights, a lot of companies would lose a lot of business.

Eating Disorders as Social Problems

The social nature of the problems of food abuse and weight obsession may not seem readily apparent. After all, most of us are used to viewing overeating as a "personal" problem, and indeed, many scientists have formulated theories about the psychological factors tied to obesity. These theories blame the eating problems solely on the individuals who manifest these problems. As a result, many people suffer from feelings of guilt and worthlessness as well as from eating problems.

Blaming the victim leads to the formulation of countless therapies diets that attempt to change the individual without changing the environment. Most of these treatments promise quick results, but when they are studied they are found to provide, at best, temporary weight loss for the vast majority of people that try them. So, while some people lose weight from fad diets or psychological therapies, many do not. Most of those who do lose weight soon regain it and begin again their search for help. It is time to realize that eating disorders and weight obsessions are not simply problems of individuals, they are problems of our society, and the only way to effectively fight them is to make changes in the the society, including changes in the American Food System.

Individual differences, of course, play a role in producing eating and weight problems. We all know that among groups of people raised and living in similar circumstances, some will develop eating problems while others will not. But theories about the causes of problem eating that focus solely on individual differences between people cannot explain why so many people have eating problems; why government surveys show that the extent of these problems is increasing,[18] and why the problem of obesity is worse in the United States than in most other countries.[19] Those people who explain this last finding as due to "abundance" cannot explain why obesity is much more common (in some studies five to seven times as prevalent) among lower-class women than among upper-class women.[20]

Psychological problems are rooted in the conditions under which we live and in the experiences we have while growing up. Some of these problems are shared by people from similar cultures, countries, and social classes, which should lead us to focus much of our attention on the social and environmental factors that produce them.

What does it mean to treat obsessions with weight, obesity, and problem eating as social, rather than as just individual problems? It means first that we must stop being so judgmental about people—including ourselves—who have these problems. They (or we) are not sinners or weaklings or selfish gluttons who deserve their fate, but people who manifest common symptoms of modern American society. This does not mean that we abrogate all responsibility for our eating problems; we are not just puppets completely at the mercy of an omnipotent society. But, if we really want to solve the problems, we must focus on the role played by the environment and the social/economic system in producing the problems.

Changing Our Environment

In order to permanently deal with our eating disorders we will have to change our environments as well as ourselves. But the problems are not simple. The society will not change overnight and the social, cultural, and economic forces that promote weight obsessions and eating disorders are too powerful to be defeated by individuals working alone. People with eating disorders and weight obsessions, and women in particular, might form support groups to share insights, feelings, and discussions about the problems. These discussions may deal with how the group members feel about their bodies, in what situations they have eating problems, how they are treated by men, children, and other women, and how they resolve the problems of food preparation. The forces promoting profit and those promoting the status quo for women are powerful and insidious. They have affected all of us. People need to share experiences if they are ever to understand that their problems are not located solely within themselves, and they need social support if they are going to try to resist these forces. The support and the sharing of experiences can come from groups of people who have been working together to solve their problems and who have come to trust one another.

But the groups cannot work only on self-education and support, as important as these tasks are. They must also work to educate others. If friends, spouses, and children maintain their old ideas about what is good to eat, how women should look, and who should buy, cook and serve food, no amount of self-understanding will be enough to allow women to combat their weight obsessions and eating disorders. The fight to change these ideas must go on in the home, in the school, and in the community. The support groups must work to provide better nutrition education in the schools in order to prevent more people from becoming overweight and to minimize the junk food brought into homes at the request of children.

The groups must also try to give people a better understanding of the social forces promoting weight obsessions and eating disorders. The methods will vary from health fairs and nutrition picnics to marathon discussions about women, bodies, and eating involving the families of group members. The resistance to these efforts will be high, but their payoff can be great, for only when the family and friends of weight-obsessed and eating-disordered people begin to fight the forces promoting these problems, rather than being part of these forces, will any permanent attack on the problems be possible.

The changes will have to include behavior as well as attitudes. When food purchasing and preparation are shared, women will be able to pay less attention to food. Even a child can learn to buy vegetables and prepare simple dishes. Some members of support groups may even be able to share food-related tasks among investment, they have avoided paying taxes on the money for four children from three or four families can eat dinner at one home one Mondays, at another home on Tuesdays, and so on.

Finally, even local social changes will not be enough. As long as the food companies continue to abuse advertising, to promote processing, to use manipulative marketing techniques, to fill vending machines with junk food, to destroy trace minerals in crops, and to portray women as either slim sex goddesses or happy homemakers dishing out dinner, weight obsessions and eating disorders will continue to be major concerns of Americans. The ongoing battles to change the food system that are described throughout this book are part of a war not only on health, nutrition, tasty food, and low prices, but also against weight obsessions, obesity, and the other eating disorders.

By this point, people who are used to reading books that promise that weight will disappear and life will be good in three weeks may be discouraged. But those books appear regularly, almost as if they were reproducing themselves—Stillman begat Atkins begat Scarsdale begat Beverly Hills—with no dent being made into the problem of eating disorders. The authors of these books focus on the effect of eating on weight, but not on the effect of social, cultural, and economic forces on eating. As a result, while they may help a handful of people to lose weight, they also reinforce the feelings of failure and self-blame felt by many other people. Since they do not deal with the root causes of eating disorders, they do not really help people to take satisfaction in their bodies or to maintain the weight loss, and they are nearly useless in preventing eating disorders from developing in children and in future generations. A social-cultural-economic-political view of eating may not promise miracle overnight cures but it does offer new feelings of pride and healthy outrage, and an opportunity to engage in a way to permanently minimize weight obsessions and eating disorders.

The Dairy Story II

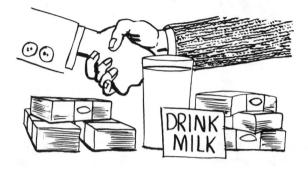

The most publicized example of agribusiness generosity toward politicians involved the dairy industry. Early in 1971, the industry requested an increase in the price guaranteed by the government for the raw milk used in many dairy products. Due to concern about large milk surpluses building up, and because the increase would raise food prices, Secretary of Agriculture Clifford Hardin announced on March 12, 1972 that the price would remain stable.

Within a week, a bill that would have bypassed the USDA and raised the price of milk was drafted by the industry and introduced in the Congress. Among the cosponsors of the bill were fifty members of the House of Representatives and eight Senators who had received campaign contributions from the dairy industry.

But the bill was not necessary, for on March 22 Richard Nixon's campaign fund received a $35,000 down payment from the industry. On March 23, industry representatives met with President Nixon. On March 25, Secretary Hardin announced the price increase, which went into effect on April Fools day. On April 5, Nixon received $45,000 more.

Between election day 1972 and May 31, 1974, one out of every seven members of Congress had received contributions from the dairy industry. But, in 1974 some of these contributions were declared illegal. The American Milk Producers Inc. was fined and two of its representatives went to jail. The story has a happy ending though. In 1976, the dairy industry spent $1.4 million on campaign contributions, more than any group other than the American Medical Association, including $11,000 for Jimmy Carter.

Based on information taken from Mark Green, *Who Runs Congress?* New York: Bantam, 1979, pp.14-17.

The Role of the Government

American industrial food production and marketing methods provide ample opportunity for food to become adulterated or overpriced, for consumers to be misled, for family farmers to be taken advantage of, and for needy people to go hungry. Although individuals can take some steps to prevent these occurrences, only when they are organized in large numbers can they collect enough resources—money, people, expertise—to do all that is necessary to obtain inexpensive, healthy foods. The most powerful of these groups organized to protect people is the federal government. Unfortunately, agribusiness uses its wealth to exert tremendous influence over government decisions regarding food.

Nowadays it takes a lot of money to successfully run a political campaign. In the 1980 Congressional elections, business political action committees (PACs) contributed over $4 million to the campaigns of fifty-four key members of Congress, accounting for two-thirds of the campaign contributions of all PACs combined.[1] Robert Dole, the Republican head of the Senate Finance Committee, received about $250,000 from business. Dan Rostenkowski, the Democratic head of the House Ways and Means Committee, received over $100,000.

Agribusiness gives more than its share. The late Ray Kroc, former chairman of the board of McDonalds, donated over $200,000 to Richard Nixon's campaign fund.[2] The dairy industry was also very generous to President Nixon, and as the Dairy Story II demonstrates, generosity of this magnitude often purchases influence.

Who Are the Regulators?

A close look at the employment histories of the people that determine government policy reveals yet another mode of industry influence. Many officials come to government agencies from industries that deal with those agencies, or go to those industries after their government service. The agencies often claim that this is the only way to attract qualified people. They maintain, with some justification, that nobody better understands the workings of an industry than a person who has worked in that industry.

The problem, of course, is conflict of interest. People who come from a regulated industry are apt to have continuing connections and loyalties within that industry and, perhaps, will be sympathetic to the needs of the industry at the expense of the needs of the public. Similarly, people who may be expecting to get jobs in an industry after leaving the government may try to avoid handing down rulings that anger or disappoint their potential employers. When the Center for Science in the Public Interest petitioned the USDA to reduce the level of nitrosamines allowed in processed meat, the request was denied by a man who, within a few months, became the president of the American Meat Institute, an industry lobbying organization.[3]

Ex-government officials working for industry can use the connections and information they gained, at taxpayer expense, to obtain advantages for the companies that hire them. In the early 1970s, when a problem arose about Red Dye #2, one of the men sent by the food industry to talk to the FDA about the problem was the former head of the colors division of that agency.[4] And in the early 1980s, Beatrice Foods had ex-Vice President Walter Mondale, a counsel in its Washington law firm, to attend to problems it had in its dealings with the government.[5]

When Clarence Palmby left his post as Assistant Secretary of Agriculture for International Affairs in charge of export programs to become a vice president at Continental Grain, he was replaced by Carole Brunthaver, from Cook Industries, another giant grain firm.[6] When Clifford Hardin resigned his position as Secretary of Agriculture and became Vice Chairman of Ralston Purina, his replacement, Earl Butz, stepped down from the boards of directors of a number of firms, including Ralston-Purina.[7]

In 1975, the FDA provided statistics on the number of senior agency officials who had come from or gone to regulated industries. One-fifth of the officials who left the agency went to work for firms regulated by the agency, and over one-forth of the officials who were still at the agency had worked at some time in a regulated firm.[8]

A sampling of FDA officials who left the agency during the Carter administration includes: Deputy Commissioner James Grant, who went to work for CPC International, a producer of margarine and peanut butter; Associate Chief Counsel for Enforcement, Richard Silverman, who went to R.J. Reynolds, producer of

Chun King Chinese Food and Hawaiian Punch, as well as ciga-
rettes; Deputy Commissioner Sherwin Gardner, who went to the
Grocery Manufacturers of America; Director of Nutrition, Ogden
Johnson, who went to the Hershey Candy Company; Director of the
Bureau of Foods, Virgil Wodicka, who came to the FDA from Hunt-
Wesson, Libby, McNeil & Libby, and Ralston-Purina, and left the
agency to become an industry consultant; and, Acting Director of
the Bureau of Foods, Howard Roberts, who came from the National
Canners Association and went to the National Soft Drink Associa-
tion.[9]

Limiting Enforcement

If these modes of influence fail and a ruling is handed down that
restricts corporate profits, the corporations can work to limit the
enforcement of the law. When consumers win a political or legal
battle they move on to new issues. Corporate representatives
remain to oversee, so to speak, the process of enforcement. They
can delay this process by means of appeals and by asking for further
study, all the while continuing the practice under dispute. They
can find loopholes or create them.

In an attempt to support family farmers, for example, a 1902
federal reclamation act limited to 160 acres the size of farms eligible
to receive government-subsidized water from federal irrigation
projects.[10] In 1933, subsidized water became available in California's Imperial Valley, which contains land that is very fertile, but
only when irrigated. To obtain access to the cheap water, large
landowners, represented by an organization called the Imperial
Irrigation District (IID), took action. They convinced Northcutt
Ely, an Assistant Secretary in the Department of the Interior, to
write a letter of exemption to the acreage limitation. Two weeks
later, Ely went to work for the IID. Not until 1963 was this letter
declared to be "clearly wrong" and the exemption overturned.
Since that time, the landowners have fought enforcement of the
law in Congress and in the courts, all of the while ignoring the
acreage limitation. As a result, a law passed in 1902 has never been
strictly enforced.

Government agencies that enact policies in the public interest
that limit corporate profits soon learn whose interest is really
important. This lesson is clearly demonstrated by the history of the
Federal Trade Commission.

The FTC was created at the turn of the century when big
business in America was subject to attacks by muckrakers,
socialists, and spokespeople for small business. To deal with these

attacks, as well as to moderate cutthroat competition and to simplify the confusing welter of state regulations, representatives of big business suggested a federal agency to regulate trade.

It may seem surprising that industrialists would want a regulatory agency, but having observed the effective connections between business and government developed by Bismarck in Germany, and feeling threatened by what the courts might do in enforcing the recently passed Sherman Antitrust Act, some corporate leaders probably felt that such an agency would be easy to control and would provide more protection than threat. In 1914, a bill was passed creating the Federal Trade Commission. The bill greatly resembled one proposed by the National Civic Federation, whose members included representatives of U.S. Steel, J.P. Morgan & Co., and other large corporations and banking firms.

The hopes of the industrialists for an easy-to-control agency were realized. So much so, that in 1938, food, drug, and cosmetic advertisers, afraid of being tightly regulated by the FDA, fought for and won the right to be regulated instead by the FTC. But when Richard Nixon appointed Miles Kirkpatrick to head the Commission, it began to become more active. The activism reached its peak under Chairman Michael Pertschuk, appointed by Jimmy Carter, with investigations and proposals that antagonized such powerful interests as the top auto manufacturers, the AMA, and the insurance industry as well as funeral directors, used car dealers, and agricultural cooperatives.

Ironically, the investigation that created the greatest furor was carried out under the power to regulate the advertising of food, drugs, and cosmetics that had been granted, in order to circumvent the FDA, in 1938. As you saw in chapter 6, advertisers, particularly those of sweets and cereals, use ads on children's television shows to gain access to an audience too young to understand the manipulations being employed. The FTC considered this to be an example of "unfair or deceptive" advertising, which it had the power to prohibit. The possibility that the commission would greatly restrict, and perhaps even ban, this practice worried all companies that rely on advertising to maximize profits. Many of them joined with the industries directly threatened by the FTC in a crusade against the agency led by the National Association of Broadcasters.

Members of Congress began to hear from these powerful interests. Soon the FTC's budget was cut, Congress took the power to veto its rulings, and its regulatory authority over advertising was limited to ads that are "false and deceptive" rather than "unfair or deceptive" as was previously the law. Subsequently, the investigation into children's advertising was dropped.

Inadequate Resources

The corporate power exhibited in this conflict with the FTC leads many government agencies to try to avoid antagonizing members of industry, for agencies lack the resources necessary for combatting powerful industries. Such has recently been the case with the Food and Drug Administration.

One major responsibility of the FDA is minimizing the presence in food of incidental additives; the dirt, bugs, poisons, and mold that enter the food supply accidentally. Many organizations, including the Consumer's Union, the U.S. General Accounting Office, the House Subcommittee on Oversight and Investigation, and the U.S. Office of Technology Assessment, have criticized the performance of the FDA in regulating these incidental additives.

The problems start with the tolerance levels for incidental additives that are set by the agency. These are the levels of contaminants that must be exceeded before the FDA takes steps to remove the food from the market. A chocolate bar can have up to three rodent hairs in a three and one-half ounce (100 gram) sample. In each can of peaches, approximately one out of twenty-one peaches can be wormy or moldy. And a can of tomato paste can contain twenty-nine Drosophila fly eggs for each three and one-half ounces and still remain on sale.[11] The tolerance levels are used because it is very difficult to produce food with no contamination, but according to Dr. J. Verret, a scientist formerly with the FDA, the levels are not in line with the current capability of food processors to produce uncontaminated food.[12] Some food manufacturers insist on products that are much cleaner than the FDA tolerances and have no trouble getting them.

The FDA is supposed to inspect food producing factories to see that sanitary manufacturing practices are maintained. But with few inspectors to police thousands of factories, each factory can be inspected only once every few years. As a result, many factory managers place low priority on sanitation. In 1970, FDA officials conducted unplanned inspections of twenty-one Kansas City warehouses as part of a training exercise for Nebraska State inspectors. Over three-quarters of the firms were found to be in violation of FDA rules.[13] More than ten tons of food that would have been marketed but for the accidental inspections was destroyed due to rodent, bird, and insect contamination. In order to evaluate the

FDA inspection program, the General Accounting Office sent auditors to ninety-seven factories selected at random. Fewer than one-third of the factories met the FDA standards.[14]

The corporations often complain of government bureaucracy and inefficiency. These complaints are not completely false. Sometimes inefficiency and the diffusion of responsibility among many agencies does slow down and complicate the regulatory process. During the last decade, at least three publicized incidents of food contamination have occurred—in Michigan in 1973, in the James River in 1975, and in the Western states in 1979—wherein contaminants were not discovered until exposure was widespread.[15]

In the 1979 incident, a power transformer in a packing plant in Billings, Montana leaked poisonous polychlorinated biphenyls (PCBs) into animal wastes that were eventually rendered into animal feed that was sold in at least nine states. Due to the vacation of an inspection official as well as delays in testing a sample from a Utah poultry plant, and more delays in notifying USDA, FDA, and state health officials, the contamination was not made public until two months after the sample was collected, which occurred who knows how long after the contamination had begun. During the investigation of the incident, officials of the USDA, the FDA, the Environmental Protection Agency, the Occupational Safety and Health Agency, the National Institute of Occupational Safety and Health, the Center for Disease Control, and three state agencies became involved. The amount of contaminated food consumed as a result of each of these major incidents is unknown.[16]

Limiting the Role of Government

But the answer to government inefficiency is not always to limit the role of the government. Contamination in food would not be reduced by cutting back even further on inspection. Sometimes the answer is to increase the power of some agencies while eliminating overlapping jurisdictions and making the agencies more answerable to the public. How many organizations can you think of that become more efficient as they are weakened?

Besides, while governments can at times be quite inefficient, they can also be quite efficient. State liquor stores and public utilities often perform more efficiently than privately owned enterprises. In fact, one of the reasons that enterprises owned by the government seem so inefficient is that the government is often forced to take over industries, such as some passenger rail lines, that are essential but that have become unprofitable and run down in the hands of business. Private industry saves the profitable businesses, such as freight rail lines, for itself. This allows the industries to take advantage of the necessary services at government expense, while pointing to the inefficiencies of the government. Appearances would be very different if the government ran the freight lines and corporations ran all of the passenger lines. In other countries, many of the most efficient enterprises are state run. We are being duped by corporate propaganda when we automatically associate government with inefficiency and industry with efficiency.

We are also being duped when we are led to believe that all government regulation is expensive. In the process of producing goods, industries also often produce social costs, such as environmental destruction or health problems in workers and consumers. Sometimes the industries are asked by government regulators to pay some of these costs. Because highly concentrated industries are able to pass on much of their expenses to consumers in the form of increased prices, they can claim that the outlays that they must make to meet government regulations are expensive to consumers.

But somebody always pays these costs. If it is not the industries that pay then it will be the workers who pay in the form of injuries, disease, loss of income, and death, or the consumers who pay in the form of increased illness and medical costs and decreased quality of life due to pollution and environmental decay. The answer is not to decrease government regulation, forcing the workers and consumers to pay all of the costs, but to force the industries to pay from their profits without passing on the payment to consumers. It makes no sense to allow processes that produce massive social costs to be highly profitable.

Furthermore, despite industry complaints of government interference, American business would be much less profitable were it not for the services rendered by the government, a fact which many corporate representatives admit to one another. Among other activities beneficial to industry, the government builds roads, ports, and airports, prosecutes thieves, issues patents, treats sewage, educates employees, subsidizes research, and opens foreign markets. In the words of a report on farm policy by the Committee for Economic Development, an organization composed primarily of the presidents and board chairmen of major corporations, big business wants to use "...positive government action...to achieve what the laissez faire approach would ordinarily expect to achieve but to do it more quickly and with less deep and protracted loss of income to the persons involved than might result if no assistance were given."[17] So it seems that many corporate executives believe that government action can, at times, be more efficient than the free market. Does this mean that the government only becomes inefficient when its actions limit corporate profits?

Paying for the government

Although they receive many benefits from government programs, corporations and their wealthy investors are not interested in paying much for these services. They use their political influence and their access to legal expertise to avoid paying their fair share of taxes. Current U.S. tax law allows people who invest in developing farmland, some orchard crops, or animal feedlots to deduct the costs of these investments from their current taxable income. Investors can delay paying taxes until the investment is sold, which is equivalent to getting an interest-free loan from the government. The returns on the investment are taxed at capital gains rates, which are often lower than income tax rates.

So, if investors in the 60 percent tax bracket invest $10,000 in cattle feedlot in 1981, they can save the $6,000 they would have paid in taxes on that money that year. If they sell their shares in the feedlot for $10,000 in 1985, they must pay a capital gains tax of 24 percent, which comes to $2,400. Even if they only break even on the investment, they have avoided paying taxes on the money for 4 years and then saved $3,600 by paying taxes at the capital gains rate rather than at the income tax rate. They can make even more of a killing by borrowing money, using their investment as collateral, and then investing the money in some profitable enterprise.

In order to take advantage of this scheme, a person needs cash, detailed knowledge of the tax laws (or the ability to hire someone with such knowledge), and a large income against which to charge off the current expenses. In other words, he or she needs to be wealthy. In 1961, Tenneco received a tax credit from farming of $13.2 million.[18]

Since the tax advantages are large when the schemes lose money, these shelters promote inefficiency. In 1972, the National Planning Association noted that taxpayers with under $50,000 adjusted gross income showed farm profits that were three times as high as their losses, while those with over $500,000 adjusted gross income showed losses which were seven times as high as their profits.[19] In 1966, 108 individuals with an annual income of over $1 million were involved in some farming in California; ninety-three of these individuals, including Ronald Reagan, reported farming losses on their income tax return.[20]

As a result of tax shelters and other tax breaks given to big business, corporate income taxes, which accounted for 23 percent of total income taxes in 1960, will account for only 7 percent by 1986.[21] And the lower the share of the corporations, the higher the share of individual taxpayers. Spokespeople for industry do not like to admit it, but programs that result in the government collecting less money in taxes have the same effect as programs that necessitate government spending, for spending more or earning less eventually come to the same thing. If we really want to cut down on government bureaucracy and lower the budget deficit, we would do better to eliminate the complex tax laws that cost the federal government $266.3 billion in these "tax expenditures" in 1982 than to destroy the FTC or the food stamp program.[22] Tax breaks that are supposed to improve the U.S. economy are really welfare for the wealthy.

Food Aid

Thus, many government policies that are justified in terms of the good of the U.S. economy turn out, upon closer examination, to be beneficial to corporate interests and investors at the expense of other people. Nowhere is this contradiction between the appearance of the goal of a government program and the actual results of that program stronger than in the American policy on food aid to underdeveloped nations. Certainly a strong humanitarian impulse lies behind some U.S. food aid. But a closer look at the Food for Peace program reveals that, here too, economic and political self-interest prevail.

The program began in the early 1950s when government supplies of surplus grain became much too large. An economy that relies on the workings of the marketplace to make decisions can be quite chaotic. Suppose, for example, that in 1985 the price of kumquats is high. Noting this, 5,000 farmers plant kumquat trees. If the trees take five years to mature, in 1990 there will be a kumquat glut on the market. The price of kumquats will drop drastically, and with it the income of the farmers. Adding to the problem, where food is grown primarily for profit only people who can afford to purchase it can be counted as consumers. So in this example, the overproduction problem would not be solved by the existence of a million people who need some additional kumquats in their diet, unless they could afford to pay for them.

Mechanisms such as this one have created U.S. farm surpluses in the midst of hunger throughout most of the twentieth century. Much U.S. farm policy has dealt with this problem of "overproduction." In 1933, the Commodity Credit Corporation was formed. The CCC loaned money to farmers who used their crops as collateral. If the market price of the crop fell below the loan rate, the farmers could forfeit on the loan, in effect selling the crop to the government. Thus, the price received by the farmers could never fall below the loan rate, which was set to equal a fair price for the crop.

After a while government stocks became excessive. The crops could not be sold without bringing down prices. One solution to the problem was to pay farmers for not planting acreage with certain crops. The irrationality of the U.S. system of growing and distributing food is clear in this program in which farmers were paid not to grow food while some people in this country, and many others throughout the world, went hungry.

A more humane solution to the surplus problem originated with the American Farm Bureau, which represents farmers of large and medium-sized farms. The bureau came up with the idea of allowing needy countries to buy grain with their local currencies. This would increase sales while keeping prices stable in the market of nations paying in dollars. In addition, in the words of a former coordinator of U.S. Food Aid, Robert R. Spitzer, "There were other people who realized that there was a great potential for the products of the American agricultural community, and that perhaps by wisely placing some of these foods in certain countries, we would develop buyers for future commodities."[23]

So, partly to feed hungry people, but mostly to get rid of surplus food while creating new markets, Public Law (PL) 480 created the Food for Peace program. Most food aid in this program is not given away. Title 1 of PL 480, which has accounted for about three-quarters of the aid given under the law, provides for long term, low-interest loans of U.S. dollars to allow foreign governments to purchase U.S. commodities. The governments sell these commodities and (until 1971) were allowed to repay the loans in the local currency generated by the sales.

According to a former Deputy Administrator of U.S. AID, "an important objective is to...insure that foreign private investment, particularly from the United States, is welcomed and well treated."[24] So in 1957, the law was changed to allow for some of the local currency generated by the sales of food to be loaned at very low interest rates to U.S. corporations to expand operations in the host countries. Two million dollars was loaned to Chase Manhattan Corporation for business development in Korea, almost $800,000 went to Coca Cola for expansion of a plant in Egypt, $200,000 aided the construction of a Gillette razor plant in Colombia, over $900,000 helped ITT put up a hotel in Tunisia, and $1 million was used by RCA for the development in Israel of a Hertz fleet.[25]

Being innovative, American policy makers have found additional uses for the money generated by PL 480. As the exact amount of these funds given to a country does not have to be approved by Congress, Food for Peace became a tool used by the State Department and the National Security Council to support military allies. Between 1968 and 1973, South Vietnam received twenty times as much food aid as five African nations that were suffering from a drought-induced famine.[26] In 1974, South Vietnam, Cambodia, Jordan, and Israel—none of which were among the most needy nations at the time—received half of the wheat, two-thirds of the animal feedstuff cereals, and all of the rice given as aid.[27] When limitations were placed by Congress on economic aid to Indochina or to Chile, food aid took up the slack.

The aid buys the cooperation of key nations. It also keeps them dependent on the United States by undermining local agricultural production. The sale of over a million tons of wheat given to the government of Colombia as aid caused the price of Colombian wheat to drop 50 percent, pushing many farmers out of business.[28] Before the aid arrived, Colombia produced three times as much wheat as it imported. After sixteen years of aid, Colombia produced less than one-eighth as much wheat as it imported. Undermining local agricultural production would appear to be a counterproductive use of aid, if it were really meant to feed people. But, in the words of the late Senator Hubert Humphrey, "...if you are looking for a way to get people to lean on you and to be dependent on you...it seems to me that food dependence would be terrific."[29]

The rulers that the government tends to support with aid are usually those that are most helpful to American business interests. When Salvadore Allende was elected President of Chile and threatened the control of Chilean resources by U.S. corporations, food aid declined to almost nothing. But, when a military junta staged a coup (with help from the United States), killed Allende, and took over the country, Chile became one of the largest recipients. To most Americans seriously concerned with helping the needy, this use of aid must seem abhorrent. But it is quite logical to many policy makers. In the words of Richard Ellerman, a former member of the National Security Council. "To give food aid to countries just because people are starving is a pretty weak reason."[30]

All of this does not mean that the United States government cannot play an important role in promoting the consumption of good food. Some hungry people have been fed with U.S. food aid. Many public officials do fight hard for consumers. The food corporations are not all-powerful. They make mistakes and some-times they even counteract one another. The margarine producers fight the butter producers. The owners of large farms sometimes fight the processors.

Sometimes the interests of businesses overlap with those of people with less power. When the food stamp program was proposed, people who wanted to fight hunger in the U.S. joined with farmers interested in ridding themselves of surplus commodities to support the program. Later, when the farmers found that exporting their crops overseas was even more profitable, the supermarket owners came to the defense of the food stamp program. As a result, many people who had been starving were able to feed themselves and their families (albeit poorly), at least until Reaganomics began its attack on the program.

Democracy is one of the great advances in the history of government. It gives the citizens of this country much more potential power in deciding the shape that their society, and hence their lives, will take. Organizations like the Center for Science in the Public Interest and the Community Nutrition Institute lobby government agencies to protect consumer interests and publish newsletters that keep people abreast of government actions that influence our diet. When the public is informed enough about a problem to get worked up about it, politicians, fearing for their jobs, may act. We did get a labeling law, albeit a weak one. Processors are sometimes caught using unsanitary practices. Some giant corpo-rations are prevented from swallowing up other corporations. DDT was banned, as were some food additives. During the Depression, desperate people overcame corporate resistance to fight to create programs like Social Security and unemployment insurance. In many states people have been able to pass legislation which provides some protection against the agribusiness assault on their diet.

But, in a system where producing and marketing food can mean big money for some people, and where those people have a disproportionate share of the resources, the policy makers will tend to be disproportionately influenced by them and the government will be run more to provide increased profits for agribusiness than to provide inexpensive, tasty, nutritious food to the rest of us. It is naive to rely on the protection of "one person-one vote" when representatives of industry have so much wealth to use in influencing government actions. In this democracy, does your voice carry as much weight as a dairy executive?

The way to take advantage of our democracy and to obtain good cheap food is not to cut back on most government regulations, thus giving even freer reign to corporate profiteers. The best way is to work toward an economic democracy, in which the control of wealth is more democratically distributed, and which would work hand in hand with our political democracy to equalize influence over decision making. The two models to avoid are a government that is not answerable to all of the people because its members are not more democratically elected, and a government that is not answerable to all of the people because it is too weak to stand up to those who control much of the wealth. The U.S. is in a position to move to a model of government that is better than either of these, but only if some social, political, and economic changes are made. If the changes are not made, the diets and lives not only of Americans but of many other people throughout the world, will continue to suffer.

The Soybean Story

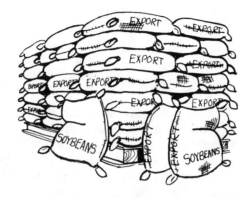

Meat in Brazil used to be cheap enough so that even peasants could regularly supplement their staple diet of black beans with beef. But when the Brazilian junta took over it was eager to increase export sales. The generals found that conditions in Brazil were excellent for growing soybeans, to be used in the developed nations for animal feed. With the help of multinational corporations, particularly from Japan and the United States, much of the land on which peasants grew corn (to feed cattle) or black beans was taken over by the Brazilian regime for the production of soybeans.

Soybeans are not part of the culture of the Brazilian peasants, they have to be processed in order to be edible, and besides they were never meant for poor Brazilians. As a result of the growth in soybean production the corporations and the junta are making big profits, but, in the early 1970s the price of land jumped over sixfold, the price of meat increased 60 percent, and not only did the price of black beans increase almost threefold, but the beans became so scarce as to necessitate rationing in the large cities. The consequences of creating a soybean export industry in Brazil, according to the French Government Center for External Trade "were that not only did a great price increase for the principal food products take place but it also became necessary to import large quantities of foodstuffs."

Based on information taken from Susan George, *How The Other Half Dies.* Montclair: Allanheld, Osmun, 1977, p. 69.

World Hunger

One of the horrible ironies of the twentieth century is the coexistence of overeating in the United States and hunger and malnutrition throughout the world, including the U.S. Definitions of malnutrition vary and so do estimates of the extent of world hunger. Some sources estimate that one out of every eight people in the world is malnourished, while others believe that as many as half of the people in the world do not get enough to eat.[1] Malnutrition produces extremely high rates of infant mortality and short life expectancies in underdeveloped nations. The proportion of babies that die before reaching their first birthday is from nine to twenty times as high in Guatemala, Indonesia, or South Africa as it is in Sweden.[2] The average Canadian can expect to live for 74 years, whereas the average Haitian or Pakistani can expect to live only to the age of 51.[3]

World hunger does not result simply from a lack of food. In 1877, four million people died in a famine in India. During World War II, Japan conquered Burma, the source of rice for the Bengal region of India, precipitating a famine during which one and a half million people died. Between 1971-1974, in the Sahel region of Africa just below the Sahara desert, drought-induced famine killed millions. The most horrifying aspect of these famines was that in the midst of all of them food continued to be exported from the starving countries, sometimes at record levels. In 1971, the first full year of the Sahel drought, over 200 million pounds of cattle were exported, along with fifty-six million pounds of fish, and thirty-two million pounds of vegetables.[4]

To understand the causes of world hunger we must understand the forces that lead to the export of food from starving nations. These forces have their roots in the European conquest of much of the world in the fifteenth through the nineteenth centuries. The actions of Great Britain during this period are representative of those of the other European powers.

Throughout the Middle Ages, British peasants lived on the land and produced barely enough food to feed themselves, their families, some landowning nobility, and a few clerics and artisans. But the technological and social changes that took place at the end of the feudal period opened up the possibility for the beginning of industry and of overseas trade, starting with woolen cloth and textiles. Some of the nobility and tradespeople began to sense the possibility of profit.

To make this profit they needed lots of wool and many workers. They got both by throwing the peasants off of the land and enclosing it for sheep pasturage. Many people who were displaced moved to the cities looking for work. In time, a textile industry grew and along with it came industries involving shipping, farm implements, land transportation, and housing.

The burgeoning trade economy, and the industrial economy that followed it, needed large amounts of raw materials—metals, lumber, wool and later cotton, food—as well as additional sources of labor and new markets. It obtained these through exploration and conquest. North America became a source of cotton, tobacco, corn, and grain. South America and the Caribbean became a source of metals, chemicals, and tropical food products.

Unfortunately for the conquerors, these areas had small populations to serve as laborers because many natives had died during the conquest as a result of harsh treatment or of new diseases brought in by the Europeans. In the islands of the Antilles, by the end of the sixteenth century, the millions in population had been reduced to about 15,000.[5] The labor problem was solved when Africa was made into a source of cheap slave labor.

The effects of the conquest were far reaching. When the British arrived in India the country was beginning its own transition to an industrial economy. It had the beginnings of a factory system, many artisans, and an export trade in silks, laces, embroidery, and jewelry. But the British wanted a colony not a rival. In the nineteenth century, due to British tax and price policies, the proportion of artisans in India fell by over half.[6] Tariffs were used to discourage textile manufacture so that the British textile industry could grow at the expense of that of India. English was decreed to be the only language permissible in schools, and the number of schools was reduced. The Governor of India, Robert Clive, was so oppressive that he was recalled and censored and he eventually committed suicide. His successor, Warren Hastings, was also investigated. Parliament declared that he had acted criminally, but that his crimes had been advantageous to England.[7]

In Africa millions of people were captured as slaves. Many died in the overcrowded, unsanitary ships that brought them to the new world, where they were treated like animals. Conditions were so bad for the slaves in the West Indies that the amount of work they did dropped, causing sugar income to decline. In 1737, the British Parliament sent a Special Commission to investigate the problem. In their report they said "The feeding and treatment of the slaves (418,000 Negroes as against 82,000 whites) and as a result, their working capacity leaves a great deal to be desired. Only twenty-five shillings a year is spent on feeding a slave with an estimated value of fifty pounds."[8] For the Commission, the problem with the mistreatment of the slaves was not that it was inhumane but that it was inefficient. In order to justify such inhumane treatment, the colonizers developed the rationale that Africans are inferior beings: dumb but strong, able to tolerate much pain, lazy, closer to animals than are white people. This rationale promoted the spread of racism.

America's Role

The U.S. spent most of the nineteenth century exploring and colonizing its own continent through conflicts with Britain and Spain and wars against Native American Indians and Mexico, with time out for a Civil War in which Northern industrialists fought Southern agriculturalists over who would control the economic policy of the country.

Toward the end of the nineteenth century American business interests began to look overseas. The colonization of Hawaii had begun in the middle of the century with white missionaries. Soon white planters and merchants arrived. But they could not fully exploit the islands while the Hawaiian monarchs ruled over them, so in 1893 the planters and merchants overthrew the monarchy with help from the U.S. Marines. They installed a white president, Sanford Dole. (Perhaps the last name rings a bell?)

In 1898, Hawaii was annexed by the United States, largely due to the lobbying of sugar interests who wanted duty-free access to U.S. markets, and to pressure from other business interests that felt that "our growing commerce on the Northern Pacific would be immensely benefitted by a control over Hawaii."[9] At the same time, U.S. troops were sent to take over the Philippines because, in the words of the President of the United States, William McKinley, "What we want is new markets, and as trade follows the flag, it looks very much as if we were [sic] going to have new markets."[10]

As in other colonized territories, the natives of Hawaii were pushed off of their land, became second-class citizens, and died of white people's diseases. Economic development took the form of ports for exporting pineapple and sugar, and of roads that travelled only from the plantations to the ports.

In the 1920s, an insect infestation threatened the pineapple crop.[11] As insurance, Del Monte opened up Haiti and the Philippines as pineapple exporters. In 1946, after a number of attempts, the International Longshoremen and Warehousemen's Union finally succeeded in organizing the Hawaiian sugar and pineapple workers. But not until the mid-1960s were the workers strong enough to demand decent wages, for once Hawaii became a state it was a little more difficult to use brutal terror tactics against the Hawaiians. The response of the pineapple companies was simple; rather than pay decent wages, they left. In 1950, Hawaii accounted for two-thirds of the pineapple trade. Now it accounts for one-third.

The shift in the location of pineapple production increased the level of unemployment in Hawaii and hurt the U.S. balance of payments, because money paid for pineapples now goes to the overseas subsidiaries of U.S. corporations. (Thus, the corporate flight overseas that has recently become common is one of the causes of stagflation: the simultaneous increase in unemployment and inflation.) At the same time, the people of the Philippines did not benefit from the shift.

The Philippines, with lots of good fruit-growing land owned by powerless peasants and with some friendly people in the government, was perfect for the needs of fruit companies like Del Monte. The Philippine government helped Del Monte to get around the restriction on corporate ownership of public lands. Unfortunately for the corporations, not everyone in the government was so helpful. In the summer of 1972, the Philippine Supreme Court ruled that U.S. corporations could own no more than forty percent of their Philippine subsidiaries and could not hold agricultural lands. Things looked tough for the corporations, but help was on the way. In September 1972, Ferdinand Marcos, president of the Phillippines, adjourned the Congress, declared martial law, reversed the decision of the Supreme Court, and outlawed strikes.

The way was open for the corporations. They began to control increasing amounts of land. What they could not get by persuasion, they got by force. In the words of an American priest, "They bulldozed people right off the land. Now they're using aerial sprays, harming farm animals and giving people terrible rashes."

The old pattern was repeated. The land from many small farms was concentrated into large plantations and the former farmers were forced to look for low-paying jobs in the plantations or in the cities. Philippine field workers often earn less than a dollar a day.[12] Banana workers wait unpaid when the fruit is not ready to be picked. When the fruit is ready, the workers often work twelve to sixteen hours a day for more than a week, frequently coming into contact with pesticides. All of this for less than one-fiftieth of the retail price paid for the bananas in Japan. Crops grown for export, called cash crops, continue to crowd out the staple food crops, grown to feed the local population. Estimates of the proportion of Philippine land covered by cash crops range from one-third to over half. Yet, sometimes as many as one-third of the bananas grown for export must be dumped in order to avoid a glut. According to a survey by the Banana Export Industry Foundation, over two-thirds of the children of workers on twenty Philippine banana plantations are malnourished.

But not everyone suffers. In Manila, fourteen high rise hotels, a convention center, and a cultural center have been built while over one million squatters live without sanitary facilities. To protect this new wealth, the Marcos government in 1977 allocated over $70 million for arms purchases from the United States.

The difference between the treatment of Hawaii and that of the Philippines is the difference between colonialism and neocolonialism. In the old days, when the merchants of one country wanted the resources of another country they sent in their troops, took over the country, appointed a governor, and took what they wanted. Nowadays, the process is slightly more subtle. The multinational corporations have learned to work with natives of the colonized territories. The corporations allow the elites of underdeveloped countries to become wealthy and help them to stay in power. In return, the native rulers allow the corporations to exploit the land, resources, and people of their countries and are willing to spend much of their wealth to import luxury goods, providing markets for the corporations.

Under special circumstances the colonizing country will still use force to protect its investments. When rulers with popular support threatened to take back from U.S. corporations the control of their countries' resources—as did Mossadegh in Iran and Arbenz in Guatemala in the 1950s, Castro in Cuba in the 60s, and Allende in Chile in the 70s—the United States sent the CIA to overthrow these rulers. The CIA attempts met with disaster at the Bay of Pigs in Cuba, but successfully aided the overthrow by military dictators of the legal leaders of Guatemala, Chile, and Iran. In the last sixty years, the U.S. armed forces have twice invaded the Dominican Republic: once in 1916, giving the South Puerto Rico Sugar

Company control of the Dominican sugar industry, and once in 1965, giving control of the industry to Gulf & Western.

But overt military intervention by the developed nations is not usually necessary, because the native elites do their best to control the people. In the words of Lord William Bentick, the British Governor General of India in 1929, "If security was wanting against popular tumult or revolution, I should say that the permanent settlement...has the great advantage...of having created a vast body of rich landed proprietors deeply interested in the continuance of British Dominion and having complete control over the mass of people."[13] Usually all the colonizer has a to do is to see that the rulers are supplied with money and arms.

The corporations can also use their political and financial power. In Senegal they convinced the government to declare that taxes could only be paid in cash, not in crops. Senegalese peasants were forced to stop growing basic food crops and to start growing peanuts for export in order to earn the cash. If the farmers in underdeveloped countries need money, they usually must go to the corporations or to institutions like the World Bank, which are influenced by the corporations. There are often strings attached. In 1974, the World Bank loaned $10 million to the government of Togo to be used solely for the production of coffee and cocoa.[14] As a result, the underdeveloped countries are constantly in debt, paying out in debt repayments almost as much as they receive in aid. To get a good credit rating the countries must follow policies, such as high taxes and low spending on social welfare, that hurt the poor.

Cash Crops

The corporations promote the growing of cash crops. The motivation for this practice is simple. Food that is eaten by the people that grow it, or that is used in barter, may prevent hunger, but it does not produce profit. Each time the food grown in a country can be turned into something to be bought and sold, the private profit food system grows a little. As profit is the primary goal of the system, the food that is produced will be that which can be sold to the people with the most money—coffee, bananas, and sugar for the United States, Europe, and Japan—not that which can be fed to the people with the most need—rice, corn, beans, and wheat for Asia, Africa, and Latin America.

One year, green bean prices were too low to justify shipping the green bean crop from Senegal to Europe. When asked what became of the crop, Paul Van Pelt, the director of Bud Holland, an agribusiness firm, answered "Since the Senegalese are not familiar with green beans and don't eat them we had to destroy them."[15] The soybean story also demonstrates what can happen when cash crops displace staple food crops.

Thus, much of the food grown in the starving underdeveloped countries is shipped to the developed countries. In 1976, Bangladesh exported over a half-million dollars of feedstuffs, three-quarters of a million dollars of meat, and over ten million dollars of fish and fishery products.[16] The leading food importers in the world are Japan, West Germany, and the United States.[17] In 1972, the United States imported almost half a million dollars of cut flowers and foliage grown on land in Central America that could have been used to grow food for millions of hungry people in Central American nations.[18] The prices paid to the underdeveloped countries for these unprocessed agricultural commodities are low and unstable. The money that does come into the countries goes to wealthy elites, not to the hungry majority.

The horror stories go on and on. Guatemalan Coca Cola workers are shot when they try to unionize.[19] Sugar plantation workers in the Dominican Republic are paid eight dollars a week by Gulf & Western while over half of the Dominicans may be anemic and chronically malnourished.[20] Similar stories could be told about Mexico, South Korea, Pakistan, or South Africa. In country after country, American multinational corporations get rich, along with local rulers and corporations from other developed nations, while people go hungry.

To add insult to injury, our economic system is "proven" to be the best one possible by comparing the high American standard of living with the suffering in underdeveloped countries. When the hungry people in these starving nations are forced to come begging for help, hard-headed realists like Garret Hardin ask, "Should those nations that do manage to put something aside be forced to come to the rescue each time an emergency occurs among the poor nations?"[21] And spokespeople for charitable institutions, like Alan Gregg, vice president of the Rockefeller Foundation liken the spread of humanity over the surface of the earth to the spread of cancer in the human body and declare " cancerous growths demand food but, as far as I know, they have never been cured by getting it."[22]

The hunger in underdeveloped countries is often blamed on ignorance and overpopulation. But United Nations' figures show that enough grain is grown each year to feed every person in the world an adequate amount of calories and protein.[23] When the nuts, fruits, vegetables, beans, and other foods that are grown are included, it becomes clear that there is enough food in the world for everyone. Even in the starving nation of Bangladesh, enough grain was produced in 1976 to feed everyone moderately well, about 2,600 calories per person per day.[24] These figures show that the major problem is not one of too little food or too many people, but of the unequal distribution of the food that is produced.

Perhaps the most momentous event that has ever occurred in the fight against world hunger was the Chinese Revolution. With the world's largest population, mostly illiterate peasants, exploited somewhat by the United States, but even more by Japan and the major European powers, China, in the first half of this century, may have been the scene of more hunger than had occurred in any other country in history. Children growing up in America in the 1940s and 1950s were told "Eat your vegetables. Don't you know that there are people starving in China?"

After two bloody revolutions and a war against the Japanese, the Communists took power. Whatever their problems, they have managed to end most of the worst hunger in China. The Chinese are not all well fed, but hunger has been drastically reduced. Bangladesh has replaced China as the example to finicky children.

But in much of the rest of the world the corporations continue to seek out profit using techniques like those they use in the United States: concentration of land into giant farms, contract farming, mechanization, pesticides, advertising and other manipulative marketing practices, control over education, and influence over government, and causing even greater unemployment, inflation, malnutrition, and disease than they cause in the U.S.

Hungry people throughout the world are becoming more aware of the injustice of the current system of food distribution. Just as the imperial powers of Europe eventually lost most of their empires, so, slowly but surely, the people in underdeveloped countries have begun to overthrow the corporate-backed dictators that exploit them. In Cuba, Nicaragua, Iran, and Vietnam revolutions have already occurred. In El Salvador, Guatemala, South Africa, the Philippines, and South Korea, revolutions are building. The leaders that come to power after these revolutions are not always saints, and many problems remain, for the effects of decades (and sometimes centuries) of exploitation do not disappear overnight, but the process of people taking control over their own lives has begun, and it will be difficult to stop. Only those people who understand the connection between the food and eating problems of the United States and those of the underdeveloped countries will realize that the anti-American sentiments that will be expressed during these revolutions will be directed at U.S. corporations, and the government forces that often work with these corporations, not at the American people, who are also being exploited.

Conclusion

Computer scientists use the phrase "Garbage In Garbage Out" (GIGO) to make the point that computers are not magic wands able to turn confused programming into sensible information. If you program garbage into a computer, you can expect to get garbage out of the computer. Perhaps we should use the term "Profit In Profit Out" (PIPO) to make the point that a food system based on private profit will produce just that—private profit. Cheap, tasty, healthy food will sometimes result from such a system, but as soon as profit, growth, concentration, and control come into conflict with any other needs, those other needs will be sacrificed. That is exactly what has occurred in the American Food System, and most of us are paying the price in illness, inflation, eating disorders, and undernutrition.

There are instances in which competition and the desire to make profits combine to lead producers to create new products that are high in quality and low in price. Propagandists for the system seldom miss a chance to point out these instances when they occur. But the propagandists usually fail to point out the many other instances in which the desire for profits leads not to innovation, quality, and bargains, but to manipulative marketing and advertising tricks, to the use of unhealthy chemicals and cheap, low-quality raw materials, and to the elimination of the very competition that was supposed to have made the system work in the first place.

The results of the quest for profits are tomatoes hard as auto bumpers, infants who ingest pesticide in their mothers' milk, starving people living in countries that export food to the United States, children manipulated into demanding highly-sugared junk food, grocers who prefer that we not realize what we are buying, doctors who are drug-and-surgery happy, bread that is bleached with acne medicine, women who are obsessed with their weight, workers who are robbed of their skills and of satisfaction with their jobs, and land that is losing its capacity to support crops.

143

One step in solving these problems is learning. Buy one of the books on additives listed in the appendix and learn to recognize the most dangerous chemicals used in your food. Reread chapter 4 and then make a trip to your local supermarket in order to reinforce your awareness of marketing tricks. Subscribe to *Nutrition Action* in order to keep up to date with what is being done to your food, to the newsletters and magazines referred to in chapter 8 to keep up with the latest nutrition research, and to *Science for the People* to find out how technology is being abused. Read the book *Food First* to learn in even greater detail the causes of world hunger. Get on the mailing list of the Center for Science in the Public Interest and the Institute for Food and Development Policy. Talk to other people in order to discover that your obsession with food slimness is shared.

But learning, while important, is not enough. After all, if you were being attacked, you would want to do more than recognize the tricks being used by your attacker and know how to treat the wounds resulting from the attack; you would also want to escape or fight. When the attack is coming from the American Food System there is no escape, so we have to fight, and the number of people and groups fighting the system is much larger than you know. The Institute for Food and Development Policy has published a pamphlet entitled *What Can You Do?* which describes some of the groups that are currently battling to change our food system. Others are mentioned in previous chapters of this book. Action for Children's Television fights manipulative advertising, the Center for Science in the Public Interest and the Community Nutrition Institute lobby the government in behalf of food consumers. The Environmental Defense Fund fights ecological destruction, Ralph Nader's Public Interest Groups and the other Nader organizations fight for consumers' rights. Farmers groups like the American Agricultural Movement are beginning to join with labor unions to fight to save family farms from bank foreclosures and corporate manipulation. Migrant farmworkers are joining unions and entering coalitions like the Farm Labor Organizing Committee. Oxfam works to help people in Third World nations feed themselves. And many women's groups have come together to fight the sexism that leads to eating disorders and body obsessions.

As long as people must rely for their food on a small number of powerful corporations whose sole motivation is to make profit, the situation will keep getting worse. The problems cannot be eliminated without attacking them at their root—the private profit food system. Sooner or later we must take the massive amount of power and resources out of the hands of the corporations and place them under democratic control. An economic democracy must join our political democracy.

Some readers will react "But isn't that socialism?" If it is, so what? I find it peculiar that while many of the thinkers who are greatly respected by Americans, and many of the countries that are our closest allies, have considered themselves to be socialist, in the United States "socialism" is still a dirty word. These countries include France, Spain, Greece, Portugal, Sweden, Austria, perhaps Italy, and in the recent past maybe Great Britain and West Germany. The thinkers include Albert Einstein, Bertrand Russell, Jean Paul Sartre, George Bernard Shaw, H.G. Wells, Helen Keller, Oscar Wilde, Jean Luc Godard, and George Orwell.

This is not a list of recommendations. Just because some respected people believed in a particular economic system is no reason for others to do the same, and most of the countries mentioned have only instituted partial versions of socialism. The point is only that outside of the United States most people in the world believe socialism to be at least worth considering. Only in the U.S. would a typical audience be shocked, and perhaps stop listening, if a speaker began a presentation with "I'd like to discuss the possibility that most Americans might benefit if we switched to a socialist economy."

Whenever we find people who are unwilling to even listen to the substance of a proposal because they've reacted so strongly to a label, we are dealing not with common sense, rationality, and science, but with ignorance, superstition, and propaganda. I'd even suggest that since Americans pride themselves on their pragmatism and their eagerness to try new methods and new ideas, the U.S. resistance to even considering socialism as a possibility is downright un-American.

If you have considered the possibility and rejected it, was your conclusion based upon careful analysis of evidence—perhaps a detailed comparison of the quality and costs of health care in the United States with those in other industrial powers that have instituted socialized medicine, or a comparison of the amount of hunger found in poor socialist nations like China and Cuba with the amount found in poor nonsocialist nations like India and the Dominican Republic? If not, you may have responded to propaganda from a government and corporations that are deathly afraid of socialism.

The Soviet Union is often used as an example of the dangers of socialism. But Americans only get to hear bad things about the

USSR. For example, the media claims that the Soviet economic system is so inefficient that the Soviet Union has to purchase grain from the United States. They do not point out that the Soviet Union is the largest producer of wheat in the world, that the grain is fed to animals so that the Soviets can eat more meat per capita than the British and that the Soviet Union has little land that is good for farming, but it had abundant energy supplies, so the Soviet leaders have decided that it is more efficient to sell gas and oil to the West and to buy Western grain. The Soviet Union has many problems and at times deserves criticism, but how can we ever decide which socialist practices might be beneficial for most Americans if the information we receive is so slanted?

The kind of socialism that would be instituted in the United States would be very different from that instituted in underdeveloped nations like Russia in the 1920s, China in the 1950s, and Cuba in the 1960s. And socialism is no panacea. It will not be the answer to every problem. But until Americans overcome their phobia toward it, we will be unable to take control of the food system away from the few people that make so much profit off of it.

I hope that even those people who are unwilling at this time to think about this step have learned a lot from this book and that they will use the information presented here to improve their eating, for there is a great deal of improvement that can be made short of major economic changes. But I also hope that many of you have been convinced by the evidence presented here that our private profit food system has become outmoded, inefficient, and unhealthy and that it is time to begin the political, social, and educational process that will take the power out of the hands of the corporations and put it into the hands of the people who produce the food and those who buy it in order to feed themselves and their families a healthy, tasty diet.

Appendix

In addition to the works cited in the references, the following information may be of interest to people who would like to learn more about our food system and work to improve it.

Books

Related to cutting down on meat consumption:

Diet for a Small Planet written by Frances Moore Lappe and published in paperback by Ballantine and the companion volume, *Recipes for a Small Planet.*

Related to understanding the additives in processed foods:

My favorite is *Eater's Digest* written by Michael Jacobson and published in paperback by Anchor Press.

The Additives Book written by Beatrice Trum Hunter and published by Keats Publishing.

A Consumer's Dictionary of Food Additives written by Ruth Winter and published by Crown Publishers.

Related to meals that are easy and unprocessed:

Keep it Simple written by William Valentine and Frances Moore Lappe and published by Pocket Books.

Related to changing the food system:

What Can We Do? written by William Valentine and Frances Moore Lappe and published by the Institute for Food and Development Policy (address below).

Newsletters and Periodicals

Food Monitor put out by World Hunger Year has a primary emphasis on world hunger.

Nutrition Action put out by the Center for Science in the Public Interest has a primary emphasis on eating in the United States.

Science for the People put out by the organization of the same name has a primary emphasis on the uses and abuses of science and technology and often prints articles on food.

Bookstores

The mail-order catalogues put out by these stores have extensive sections on food and agriculture:

Earthwork, 3410 19th St., San Francisco, CA 94110

Food for Thought, 67 N. Pleasant St., Amherst, MA 01002

Modern Times Bookstore, 968 Valencia St., San Francisco, CA 94110

Organizations

Action for Children's Television, 46 Austin St., Newtonville, MA 02160 fights the abuse of food advertising on children's television.

The Center for Science in the Public Interest, 1501 16th St., NW, Washington D.C. 20036 puts out books, posters and periodicals dealing with eating in the United States and lobbies the U.S. Government on food issues.

The Center for the Study of Responsive Law, P.O. Box 19367, Washington D.C. 20036 is an organization founded by Ralph Nader to research, educate and lobby on consumer issues.

Institute for Food and Development Policy, 1885 Mission St., San Francisco, CA 94103 puts out books, pamphlets, and newsletters and does research and education on food issues, particularly with reference to world hunger.

International Academy of Preventive Medicine, 10950 Grandview, Suite 469, Overland Park, Kansas 60210 puts out a newsletter on nutrition and is a source of addresses for doctors who have a preventive emphasis.

Oxfam America, 115 Broadway, Boston, MA organizes efforts to fight famine and chronic hunger in developing nations.

Science for the People, 897 Main St., Cambridge, MA 02139 does research and education on the abuse of science and technology.

World Hunger Year, 350 Broadway, New York, NY 10013 deals primarily with issues of world hunger.

Footnotes

The Chicken Story

1. Frink, C.R., "More food from fewer acres." *Food and Social Policy: Occasional Papers of the Connecticut Humanities Council,* #1, 1978, p. 36.
2. Wellford, H., *Sowing the Wind.* New York: Bantam, 1973, p. 109.
3. "Chubby chickens on the rise." *Nutrition Action,* July, 1980, p. 6.
4. Mason, J. & Singer, P., *Animal Factories.* New York: Crown, 1980, pp. 42, 55.

Farming

1. Weir, D. & Shapiro, M., *Circle of Poison.* San Francisco: Institute for Food and Development Policy, 1981, p. 29.
2. January 30, 1962, cited in Mason et al., op. cit., p. 1.
3. Pimental, D., Oltenacu, P.A., Nesheim, M.C., Krammel, J., Allen, M.S. & Chick, S., "The potential for grass-fed livestock: Resource constraints." *Science,* vol. 207, February 22, 1980, p. 843.
4. Ibid., p. 844.
5. Frink, C.R., "More food from fewer acres." *The Connecticut Scholar,* Occasional Paper No. 1, 1978, p. 36.
6. Mason et al., op. cit., p. 84.
7. Green, M., *Eating Oil.* Boulder: Westview, 1978, p. 95.
8. Mason et al., op. cit., p. 58.
9. Hess, J.L. & Hess, K., *The Taste of America.* New York: Penguin, 1977, p. 43.
10. National Academy of Science study cited in Belden, J., Edwards, G., Guyer, C. & Webb, L. (Eds.), *New Directions in Farm, Land, and Food Policies.* Washington, D.C.: Conference on Alternative State and Local Policies, pp. 140, 141.
11. Fowler, C., "Sowing the seeds of destruction." *Science for the People,* September/October, 1980, p. 8.
12. Perelman, M., *Farming for Profit in a Hungry World.* New York: Universe, 1977, p. 47.
13. All information on the low quality of crops from the new seeds from p. 46.
14. Fowler, op. cit., p. 9.
15. The Coalition for Responsible Genetic Research, "Perspectives on biotechnology." *Science for the People,* September/October, 1980, p. 11.

16. Fowler, op. cit., p. 9.
17. Perelman, op. cit., p. 11.
18. Belden et al., op. cit., p. 123.
19. *Changes in Farm Production and Efficiency.* USDA Statistical Bulletin No. 612, 1977, p. 27.
20. Krenz, R.D., Heid, W.G. & Sitler, H., *Economics of Large Wheat Farms in the Great Plains.* USDA Agricultural Economic Report No. 264, July, 1974, p. 11.
21. Pimentel, D., Krammel, J., Gallahan, D., Hough, J., Merril, A., Schreiner, I., Vittum, P., Koziol, F., Back, E., Yen, D. & Fiance, S., "Benefits and costs of pesticide use in U.S. food production." *Bioscience,* vol. 28, #12, December, 1978, p. 778.
22. All information on animals killed by pesticides from van den Bosch, R., *The Pesticide Conspiracy.* Garden City: Anchor, 1980, p. 28.
23. Fellmuth, R.C., *The Politics of Land.* New York: Grossman, 1973, p. 108.
24. Wellford, H., *Sowing the Wind.* New York: Grossman, 1972, p. 213.
25. Information on chemical residues in food from Siskind, L., *The Pesticide Syndrome.* San Francisco: Earthworks, 1979, p. 31.
26. Harris, S.G. & Highland, J.H., *Birthright Denied: The Risks and Benefits of Breast-Feeding.* Washington, D.C.: Environmental Defense Fund, 1981, p. 6.
27. Information on exported pesticides from Weir et al., op. cit., pp. 4-7.
28. Ibid., p. 26.
29. Ibid., p. 31.
30. Ibid., p. 32.
31. Ibid., pp. 28, 29.
32. Siskind, op. cit.
33. Van den Bosch, op. cit., pp. 23, 24.
34. Pimental, Krammel et al., op. cit., p. 778.
35. Wellford, op. cit., p. 282.
36. Van den Bosch, op. cit., p. 157.
37. *Census of Agriculture.* Bureau of Census, 1974.
38. *Food Monitor.* September/October, 1980, p. 22.
39. Many of these studies are reviewed in Madden, J.P. & Partenheimer, E.J., "Evidence of economies and diseconomies of farm size." In G. Ball & E.O. Heady (Eds.), *Size, Structure, and Future of Farms.* Ames: Iowa State University, 1971, pp. 91-107.
40. Ibid., p. 96.
41. Hightower, J., *Eat Your Heart Out.* New York: Vintage, 1976, p. 159.
42. All information on Tenneco from Frundt, H.J., "Agribiz insignificant for nation's largest farmer." In *Agribusiness Manual.* New York: Interfaith Center for Corporate Responsibility, 1978, pp. V9-V15.
43. Information on arable land from *FAO Production Yearbook,* vol. 33, 1979.
44. Information on crop production per acre from *Agricultural Statistics.* USDA, 1976, pp. 9, 35, 42.

45. Pimental, D., Terhune, E.C., Dyson-Hudson, R., Rochereau, S., Sumis, R., Smith, E.A., Denman, D., Reifschneider, D. & Shepard, M., "Land degradation: Effects on food and energy resources." *Science,* vol. 194, October 8, 1976, p. 150.
46. Ibid., p. 151.
47. Belden et al., op. cit., p. 121.
48. Goldschmidt, W., *As You Sow.* Montclair: Allanheld Osmun, 1978, Part II.

The Tomato Story

1. Vandermeer, J., "Agricultural research and social conflict." *Science for the People,* vol. 13, #1, January/February, 1981, p. 6.
2. Information on the board of regents is taken from *Nutrition Action,* May, 1980, p. 5.
3. Taper, B., "The bittersweet harvest." *Science 80,* November, 1980, p. 81.
4. California Agrarian Action Project and Yolo Friends of the Farmworkers. "No hands touch the land: Automating California's farms." *Science for the People,* vol. 10, #1, January/February, 1978, pp. 20-28.
5. Taper, op. cit.
6. California Agrarian Action Project, op. cit.
7. Ibid., p. 23.
8. Whiteside, T., "Tomatoes." *New Yorker,* January 24, 1977, pp. 36-61.

Technology

1. Rasmussen, W.D., "The mechanization of agriculture." *Scientific American,* September, 1982, p. 77.
2. California Agrarian Action Project and Yolo Friends of the Farmworkers, op. cit., pp. 20-28.
3. Perelman, D., *Farming for Profit in a Hungry World.* New York: Universe, 1977.
4. *Statistical Abstract of the United States.* Bureau of the Census, 1979, Table #681, p. 410.
5. New York: Monthly Review, 1974.
6. Pimental, D., Hurd, L.E., Bellotti, A.C., Forster, M.J., Oka, I.N., Sholes, O.D. & Whitman, R.J., "Food production and the energy crisis." *Science,* vol. 182, November 2, 1973, pp. 443-449.
7. Steinhart, J.S. & Steinhart C.E., "Energy use in the U.S. food system." *Science,* vol. 184, April 19, 1974, pp. 307-316.
8. Pimentel et.al., op. cit.
9. Cited in Perelman, op. cit., p. 161.
10. Goetsch, C.H., "Technical change and the distribution of income in rural areas." *American Journal of Agricultural Economics,* vol. 54, May, 1972, p. 326.
11. California Agrarian Action Project et al., op. cit., p. 24.
12. Barnett, P., "The pesticide connection." *Science for the People,* vol. 12, #4, July/August, 1980, p. 8.
13. *Nutrition Action,* May, 1980, p. 5.

14. Information on CAST from "Objective science groups or industry's puppets?" *Nutrition Action,* February, 1979, p. 7 and "Scientists quit antibiotics panel at CAST," *Science,* vol. 203, February 23, 1979, pp. 732, 733.

15. "The political influence of a hard-boiled industry." *Nutrition Action,* December, 1978, p. 9.

16. "ACSH: Another objective group?" *Nutrition Action,* February, 1979, p. 12.

17. Harty, S., *Hucksters in the Classroom: A Review of Industry Propaganda in Schools.* Washington, D.C.: Center for Study of Responsive Law, 1979, p. 311.

18. Information on funds received by the Harvard Department of Nutrition from Rosenthal, B., Jacobson, M. & Bohm, M., "Professors on the take." In L. Hoffman, *The Great American Nutrition Hassle.* Palo Alto: Mayfield, 1978, pp. 379-391.

19. Information on the report on cholesterol from "Academy gets egg on its face." *Nutrition Action,* July, 1980, p. 10.

The Bread Story

1. Hall, R.H., *Food for Nought: The Decline in Nutrition.* New York: Harper & Row, 1974, pp. 19, 27.

2. Ibid.

3. Ibid., p. 262.

Processing

1. Jacobson, M., *Eater's Digest: The Consumer's Factbook of Food Additives.* Garden City: Anchor, 1976, p. 4.

2. Information on sales of vegetables and frozen foods from Jacobson, M. & Brewster, L., *The Changing American Diet.* Washington, D.C.: Center for Science in the Public Interest, 1978, pp. 50, 28.

3. LeBovit, C. & Boehm, W.T., "Changes to meet dietary goals." *National Food Review,* Fall, 1979, pp. 24, 25.

4. *Food Engineering,* vol. 43, #10, 1971, p. 5.

5. Jacobson, *Eater's Digest,* op. cit., p. 227.

6. Food and Agricultural Organization, "Toxicological evaluation of some food colors, emulsifiers, stabilizers, anti-caking agents and certain other substances." *FAO Nutritional Meetings Report Series 46A,* 1970.

7. Jacobson, op. cit., pp. 95-97.

8. *Wall Street Journal,* June 21, 1977.

9. Jacobson, op. cit., p. 71.

10. Ibid., p. 226.

11. Coconuts quote from Gussow, J.D. (Ed.), *The Feeding Web: Issues in Nutritional Ecology.* Palo Alto: Bull, 1978, p. 169.
Dairy flavors quote from *Food Technology,* vol. 31, #7, July, 1977, p. 14.

12. *Food Technology,* vol. 37, #10, October, 1979, p. 11.

13. Gussow, op. cit., p. 176.

14. *Food Product Development,* vol. 12, #9, October, 1978, p. 11.

15. Information on loss of nutrition in processed foods from Schroeder, H.A., "Losses of vitamins and trace minerals resulting from processing and preservation of foods." *American Journal of Clinical Nutrition,* May 24, 1971, pp. 562-573.

16. "Nutritional shortchanging from modern food processing." *Consumer Bulletin,* January, 1973, pp. 19-23.

17. Clydesdale, F.M., *Journal of the American Dietetic Association,* vol. 74, January, 1979, pp. 17-22.

18. Gussow, op. cit., p. 203.

19. *Food Technology,* vol. 2, February, 1977, p. 7.

20. "The vitamin game in action." *Nutrition Action,* November, 1978, p. 5.

21. Cited in Grieg, W.S., *The Economics of Food Processing.* Westport: Avi, 1971, p. 57.

22. Gussow, op. cit., p. 202.

23. Ibid.

24. Moskowitz, M., Katz, M. & Levering, R. (Eds.), *Everybody's Business.* San Francisco: Harper & Row, 1980, p. 29.

25. "The food industry monopoly causes prices to skyrocket." *Nutrition Action,* November, 1979, p. 4.

26. Information on ketchup and frosting from Moskowitz et al., op. cit., p. 31.

27. "The market function of costs for food between America's fields and tables." Economic Research Service (USDA) for the Committee on Agriculture and Forestry, U.S. Senate, March 26, 1975, p. 79.

28. "On the influence of market structure on the profit performance of food manufacturing companies." Federal Trade Commission, September, 1969.

29. USDA, op. cit.

30. Parker, R.C. & Connor, J.M., "Estimates of consumer loss due to monopoly in the U.S. food manufacturing industry." *American Journal of Agricultural Economics,* vol. 61, #4, November, 1979, p. 637.

31. Cited in Moskowitz et al., op. cit., p. 40.

32. See ibid. for many examples.

Marketing

1. Marion, D.R., Mueller, W.F., Cotterill, R.W., Geithman, F.E. & Schmelzer, J.R., *The Food Retailing Industry: Structure, Profits and Prices.* New York: Praeger, 1979, p. 1.

2. Ibid., p. 15.

3. Ibid., p. 114.

4. Ibid., p. 139.

5. Ibid., p. 68.

6. FTC, *Economic Report on Food Chain Selling Practices in the District of Columbia and San Francisco.* Prepared for the Committee on Government Operations, 91st Congress, July, 1969.

7. Cross, J., *The Supermarket Trap: The Consumer and the Food Industry.* Bloomington: Indiana University Press, 1970.
8. "Tips for productive price marking." *Progressive Grocer,* October, 1978, p. 58.
9. Taylor, P., "Packaging: The costs add up." In C. Lerza & M. Jacobson (Eds.), *Food for People Not for Profit.* New York: Ballantine, 1975, pp. 140-144.
10. Ibid.
11. Nader, R. & Moore, B., "Competition and consumer sovereignty." Ibid., pp. 130-134.
12. Gallo, A.E. & Connor, J.M., "Packaging in food marketing." *National Food Review,* Spring, 1981, p. 46.
13. Taylor, op. cit.
14. Boas, M. & Chain, S., *Big Mac: The Unauthorized Story of McDonalds.* New York: Mentor, 1976, p. 74.
15. Taylor, op. cit.
16. Cross, op. cit.
17. Ibid.
18. Devine, D.G. & Marion, B.W., "The influence of consumer price information on retail pricing and consumer behavior." *American Journal of Agricultural Economics,* vol. 61, May, 1979, pp. 228-237.
19. *Disease Prevention and Health Promotion Act of 1978.* Hearings before the Subcommittee on Human Resources, June 9, 1978.
20. Cross, op. cit.
21. Brewster, L. & Jacobson, M.F., *The Changing American Diet.* Washington, D.C.: Center for Science in the Public Interest, 1978, p. 27.
22. Jacobson, M.F., *Eater's Digest: The Consumer's Factbook of Food Additives.* Garden City: Anchor, 1976, p. 60.
23. Settle, D.M. & Patterson, C.C., "Lead in albacore: Guide to lead pollution in Americans." *Science,* vol. 207, March 14, 1980, pp. 1167-1175.
24. Jacobson, op. cit., pp. 86, 87.
25. FDA, *Consumer Nutrition Knowledge Survey Report 1,* 1973-74, p. x.
26. Connor, J.M., "Food product proliferation: Part I." *National Food Review,* Spring, 1980, p. 12.
27. FTC, op. cit., p. 30.
28. Ibid.
29. Ibid., p. 3.
30. Skelly, G.U., "Where do food stamp recipients shop for food?" *National Food Review,* Spring, 1980, p. 22.
31. Marion, D.R., "Toward revitalizing inner-city food retailing." *National Food Review,* Summer, 1982, p. 22.
32. Lindstrom, H. & Henderson, P.G., "Farmer to consumer marketing." *National Food Review,* Fall, 1979, pp. 22-23.

The Fast Food Story

1. Matsumoto, M., "The cost of 'fast food' meals at home." *National Food Review,* Summer, 1979, p. 10.

2. Storm, B., "The fast-food confrontation." *Madison Avenue,* October, 1979, p. 50.
3. Boas, M., & Chain, S., *Big Mac: The Unauthorized Story of McDonalds.* New York: Mentor, 1976, pp. 29, 30.
4. Matsumoto, op. cit., p. 73.
5. Boas et al., op. cit., p. 73.
6. *Consumer Reports,* September, 1979, p. 512.

Preparation

1. Burros, M., "The real cost of convenience foods." In C. Lerza & M. Jacobson (Eds.), *Food for People Not for Profit.* New York: Ballantine, 1975, pp. 135, 136.
2. Curtis, B., "Capital, the state and the origins of the working-class household." In B. Fox (Ed.), *Hidden in the Household.* Toronto: Women's Press, 1980, p. 12.
3. Ibid.

Advertising

1. Potter, D., *People of Plenty.* Chicago: University of Chicago Press, 1954, p. 175.
2. "Water Sports." *Madison Avenue,* October, 1979, pp. 42-48.
3. "Definition of Brooklyn man held best." *Advertising Age,* July 28, 1932, p. 1.
4. *Advertising Age,* September 10, 1981, p. 1.
5. Ibid., September 10, 1981, p. 1.
6. Barcus, F.E. & McGlaughlin, L., *Food Advertising on Children's Television.* Newtonville: Action for Children's Television, 1978, p. 7.
7. Bishop, F.D., *The Economics of Advertising.* London: Robert Hale, 1949, p. 19.
8. FTC actions are reported each year in the *Federal Register.*
9. Bottled water quotes from "Water Sports," op. cit.
10. "Snack food: From salt to nuts." *Madison Avenue,* October, 1979, p. 56.
11. Silverstein, B., Perdue, L. & Kelly, E., "The role of the mass media in promoting eating disorders among women." Unpublished manuscript.
12. Barcus et al., op. cit.
13. Gussow, J.D., "Counternutritional messages of TV ads aimed at children." In Gussow, J.D. (Ed.), *The Feeding Web: Issues in Nutritional Ecology.* Palo Alto: Bull, 1975.
14. Ward, W., Reale, G. & Levinson, D., "Children's perceptions, explanations and judgements of television advertising: A further explanation." Cited in Liebert, R., Neale, J.M., & Davison, E.S., *The Early Window: Effects of Television on Children and Youth.* New York: Pergamon, 1973, p. 130.
15. Updegraff, R.R., "Advertising to children." *Advertising and Selling,* no. 9, February, 1912, p. 120.

156   FED UP

16. Gussow, op. cit.
17. "The Idaho potato commission." *Madison Avenue,* October, 1978, p. 45.
18. *Advertising Age,* September 10, 1981, p. 125.
19. Ibid., September 6, 1979, p. 136.
20. Barcus et al., op. cit., p. 7.
21. Ibid., pp. 58, 61.
22. Technical Study No. 10, *Special Studies in Food Marketing,* June, 1966, p. 65.
23. Nader, R. & Moore, B., "Competition and consumer sovereignty." In C. Lerza & M. Jacobson (Eds.), *Food for People Not for Profit.* New York: Ballantine, 1975, p. 133.
24. *The Market Function of Costs for Food Between America's Fields and Tables.* Economic Research Service (USDA) for the Committee on Agriculture and Forestry, U.S. Senate, March 26, 1975, p. 79.
25. Gussow, op. cit.

Education

1. FDA, *Consumer Nutrition Knowledge Survey.* Report 1, 1973-74.
2. Schwartz, N.G., "Nutrition knowledge, attitudes and practices of Canadian public health nurses." *Journal of Nutrition Education,* vol. 8, #1, January-March, 1976, pp. 28-31.
3. Podell, R.N., Gary, L.R. & Keller, K., "A profile of clinical nutrition knowledge among physicians and medical students." *Journal of Medical Education,* vol. 50, September, 1975, pp. 888-892.
4. Gould Gillis, D.E. & Sabry, J.H., "Daycare teachers: Nutrition knowledge, opinions, and use of food." *Journal of Nutrition Education,* vol. 12, #4, 1980, pp. 200-204.
5. Cook, C.B., Eiler, D.A. & Kaminaka, E.C., "How much nutrition education in grades K-6?" *Journal of Nutrition Education,* vol. 9, #3, July-September, 1977, pp. 131-135.
6. *Nutrition Education in Medical Schools.* Hearing before the Subcommittee on Nutrition, Committee on Agriculture, Nutrition and Forestry, U.S. Senate, 95th Congress, second session, pt. 1, p. 108.
7. Guthrie, H.A. & Teply, C.L., "Nutrition in medical education a premedical alternative." *American Journal of Clinical Nutrition,* vol. 32, August, 1979, pp. 1557, 1558.
8. *Nutrition Education in Medical Schools,* op. cit.
9. Harty, S., *Hucksters in the Classroom: A Review of Industry Propaganda in Schools.* Washington, D.C.: Center for Study of Responsive Law, 1979, p. 8.
10. Ibid., p. 33.
11. Ibid., p. 37.
12. Barnouw, E., *Documentary.* Oxford: Oxford University Press, 1983, p. 219.
13. Packard, V.O., *The Hidden Persuaders.* New York: McKay, 1957, p. 158.

Health

1. Dreitzel, H.P. (Ed.), *The Social Organization of Health*. New York: Macmillan, 1971, p. 4.
2. *Getting Ready for National Health Insurance: Unnecessary Surgery*. Hearings before the Subcommittee on Oversight and Investigations of the Committee on Interstate and Foreign Commerce, House of Representatives, 94th Congress, first session, p. 67.
3. Illich, I., *Medical Nemesis*. New York: Random House, 1979, p. 255.
4. Weinsler, R.L., Hunker, E.M., Kramdieck, C.L., & Butterworth, C.E., "Hospital malnutrition: a prospective evaluation of general medical patients during the course of hospitalization." In *Nutrition Education in Medical Schools Pt. 1*. Hearings before the Subcommittee on Nutrition of the Committee on Agriculture, Nutrition and Forestry, U.S. Senate, 95th Congress, pp. 54-63.
5. *Statistical Abstract of the United States*. Department of the Census, 1980.
6. Sivard, R.L., *World Military and Social Expenditures*. Washington, D.C.: World Priorities, 1980.
7. *Health United States 1979*. National Center for Health Statistics, p. 117.
8. *Vital Statistics of the United States, 1978, Vol. II, Mortality, Part A*. National Center for Health Statistics.
9. *Health and Nutrition Examination Survey 1971-74*. National Center for Health Statistics, 1978.
10. *Health United States 1979*. National Center for Health Statistics, p. 31.
11. Ibid.

The Soda Pop Story

1. Information on soda pop consumption is taken from Brewster, L. & Jacobson, M., *The Changing American Diet*. Washington, D.C.: Center for Science in the Public Interest, 1978, p. 45 and Moskowitz, M., Katz, M. & Levering, R., *Everybody's Business*. San Francisco: Harper & Row, 1980, p. 66.
2. Bureau of Vital Statistics. *Vital and Health Statistics,* Series 11, #2, pp. 13, 32.
3. Brewster et al., op. cit., p. 44.
4. *Advertising Age,* op. cit., p. 1.
5. Brewster et al., op. cit., p. 45.
6. Bureau of Vital Statistics, op. cit., p. 32.

Eating Disorders

1. Van Itallie, T., *Diet related to killer diseases—Obesity*. Testimony before the Select Committee on Nutrition and Human Needs. U.S. Senate, 95th Congress, February 1 & 2, 1977.

2. Stunkard, A.J., Levine, H. & Fox., S., "The Management of obesity: Patient self-help and medical treatment." *Archives of Internal Medicine,* vol. 125, 1970, pp. 1367-1373.

3. Druss, V. & Henifin, M.S., "Why are so many anorexics women?" In R. Hubbard & M.S. Henifin (Eds.), *Women Looking at Biology Looking at Women: A Collection of Feminist Critiques.* Cambridge: Schenkman, 1979.

4. *Health United States 1978.* National Center for Health Statistics, Table 42.

5. Garner, D., Garfinkel, P.E., Schwartz, P. & Thompson, M., "The cultural pressure on women for thinness." *Psychological Reports,* vol. 47, 1980, pp. 483-491.

6. Silverstein, B., Perdue, L. & Kelly, E., "Eating disorders, gender differences, and the mass media." Unpublished manuscript, S.U.N.Y. at Stony Brook, Department of Psychology.

7. Ibid.

8. Wooley, S. & Wooley, D., "Should obesity be treated at all?" Unpublished manuscript, University of Cincinnati Medical Center.

9. Richardson, S.A., Goodman, N., Hastorf, A. & Dornbusch, S.M., "Cultural uniformity in reaction to physical disabilities." *American Sociological Review,* vol. 26, 1961, p. 241.

10. Silverstein et al., op. cit.

11. Schachter, S., "Obesity and eating." *Science,* vol. 161, 1968, p. 751.

12. Aronson, N., "Working up an appetite." In J.R. Kaplan (Ed.), *A Woman's Conflict: The Special Relationship Between Women and Food.* Englewood Cliffs: Prentice Hall, 1980.

13. Data on calories in processed versus unprocessed foods taken from Krauss, B., *Calorie Guide to Brand Name Foods.* New York: New American Library, 1981.

14. Van Itallie, T., "Dietary Fiber and obesity." *American Journal of Clinical Nutrition,* vol. 31, 1978, pp. 543-552.

15. Van Itallie, *Diet related to killer diseases—Obesity,* op cit.

16. Dwyer, J., "Sixteen popular diets: Brief nutritional analysis." In A.J. Stunkard (Ed.), *Obesity.* Philadelphia: W.B. Saunders, 1980.

17. Moskowitz, M., Katz, M. & Levering, R. (Eds.), *Everybody's Business.* San Francisco: Harper & Row, 1980, p. 41.

18. *Vital and Health Statistics,* Series 11, no. 208, pp. 5-13.

19. Christakis, G., "The prevalence of adult obesity." In G. Bray (Ed.), *Obesity in Perspective.* Fogarty International Center for Advanced Study in the Health Sciences, vol. 12, pt. 2, 1973.

20. Garn, S.M., Bailey, S.M., Cole, P.E. & Higgins, I.T.T., "Level of education, level of income and level of fatness in adults." *American Journal of Clinical Nutrition,* vol. 30, 1977, pp. 721-725.

Government

1. *In These Times,* May 6-12, 1981, p. 4.

2. Boas, M. & Chain, S., *Big Mac: The Unauthorized Story of*

McDonalds. New York: Mentor, 1976, p. 174.

3. Dumont, R. & Cohen, N., *The Growth of Hunger: Concerning a New Politics of Agriculture.* Salem, NH: Merrimack, 1980, p. 178.

4. Verret, J. & Carper, J., *Eating May Be Hazardous to Your Health.* Garden City: Anchor, 1975, p. 78.

5. Taylor, S., "Those job-hopping Carter people." *New York Times,* May 10, 1981, p. F15.

6. Krebs, A.V., "Of the grain trade, by the grain trade and for the grain trade." In C. Lerza & M. Jacobson (Eds.), *Food for People Not for Profit.* New York: Ballantine, 1975, p. 356.

7. *New York Times,* November 1, 1971, p. 1 and November 18, 1971.

8. Committee for Voluntary Regulation of the Appointment Process, *Study on Federal Regulation.* U.S. Senate, 1977.

9. FDA, "Graduates in industry." *Nutrition Action,* January, 1980, p. 7.

10. Information on the nonenforcement of the irrigation law is from *In These Times,* July 16, 1980, p. 4.

11. *The Food Defect Action Levels,* FDA, 1980.

12. Verret et al., op. cit., p. 192.

13. Turner, J.S., *The Chemical Feast.* New York: Penguin, 1976, p. 76.

14. Lucas, S., *The FDA.* Millbrae, California: Celestial Arts, 1978, p. 22.

15. "Swifter action sought on food contamination." *Science,* vol. 207, January 11, 1980, p. 163.

16. Ibid.

17. Ritchie, M., *The Loss of Our Family Farms: Inevitable Result or Conscious Policy.* 824 Shotwell, San Francisco, California, 1979.

18. Goldschmidt, W., *As You Sow.* Montclair: Allanheld Osmun, 1978, p. xxxvii.

19. Ibid.

20. Fellmuth, R.C., *Politics of Land: Ralph Nader's Study Group Report on Land Use in California.* New York: Grossman, 1973, p. 78.

21. "Why does the right own the tax issue?" Interview with Congressman Byron Dorgan. *The Village Voice,* March 30, 1982, p. 6.

22. Ibid.

23. Cited in Lappe, F.M. & Collins, J., *Food First: Beyond the Myth of Scarcity.* New York: Ballantine, 1978, p. 328.

24. George, S., *How the Other Half Dies: The Real Causes of World Hunger.* Montclair: Allanheld Osmun, 1977, p. 47.

25. Frundt, H., *Agribusiness Manual.* New York: Interfaith Center on Corporate Responsibility, pp. II-9-II-12.

26. Lappe et al., op. cit., p. 337.

27. Dumont, op. cit., p. 159.

28. Frundt, op. cit., p. II-13.

29. Cited in Lappe et al., op. cit., pp. 386, 387.

30. North American Congress on Latin America, *Latin America and Empire Report,* vol. IX, #7, October 6, 1975, p. 17.

World

1. Bernstein, B., "Preliminary readings in 'the world food problem'." *Food and Social Policy: Occasional Papers of the Connecticut Humanities Council #1,* 1978, p. 11.

2. Sivard, R.L., *World Military and Social Expenditures.* World Priorities, 1980.

3. Ibid.

4. Lappe, F.M. & Collins, J., *Food First: Beyond the Myth of Scarcity.* New York: Ballantine, 1978, pp. 94, 102.

5. De Castro, J., *The Geography of Hunger.* Boston: Little, Brown, 1952, p. 108.

6. Ibid., p. 180.

7. Ibid., p. 185.

8. Ibid., p. 118.

9. Williams, W.A., *The Roots of the American Empire.* New York: Random House, 1969, p. 441.

10. Ibid.

11. Information on the pineapple industry in Hawaii and the Philippines is taken from Burbach, R. & Flynn, P., *Agribusiness in the Americas.* New York: Monthly Review, 1980, pp. 192-205.

12. Information on the Philippine banana industry is taken from Lappe, F.M. & McCallie, E., "Banana hunger: Agribusiness in the Philippines." *Reprint Packet 1.* San Francisco: Institute for Food and Development Policy, March, 1979, pp. 7-9.

13. George, S., *How the Other Half Dies: The Real Causes of World Hunger.* Montclair: Allanheld Osmun, 1977, p. 57.

14. Dumont, R. & Cohen, N., *The Growth of Hunger: Concerning a New Politics of Agriculture.* Salem, NH: Merrimack, 1980, p. 35.

15. Lappe, F.M. & Collins, J., "Turning the desert green for international agribusiness." *Reprint Packet 1,* op. cit., p. 10.

16. FAO Trade Yearbook, 1977, vol. 31., p. 323.

17. Ibid.

18. Goldberg, R., *Agribusiness Management for Developing Countries— Latin America.* Cambridge, Mass.: Ballinger, 1974, p. 371.

19. *New York Times,* June 6, 1980.

20. Ledogar, R.J., *Hungry for Profits.* New York: IDOC/North America, 1975, pp. 80, 85.

21. Gussow, J.D., *The Feeding Web: Issues in Nutritional Ecology.* Palo Alto: Bull, 1975, p. 77.

22. Ibid., p. 78.

23. Lappe, F.M. & Collins, J., *Food First Resource Guide.* San Francisco: Institute for Food and Development Policy, 1979, p. 7.

24. Ibid.